# Training
# Your Brain
## FOR

# DUMMIES®

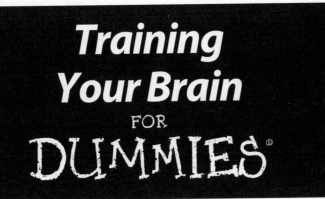

# Training Your Brain FOR DUMMIES®

by Dr Tracy Packiam Alloway
Puzzles by Timothy E. Parker

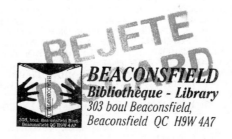

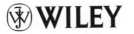

## WILEY

A John Wiley and Sons, Ltd, Publication

**Training Your Brain For Dummies®**

Published by
**John Wiley & Sons, Ltd**
The Atrium
Southern Gate
Chichester
West Sussex
PO19 8SQ
England

E-mail (for orders and customer service enquires): cs-books@wiley.co.uk

Visit our Home Page on www.wiley.com

For general information on our other products and services, please contact our Customer Care Department within the U.S. at 877-762-2974, outside the U.S. at 317-572-3993, or fax 317-572-4002.

For technical support, please visit www.wiley.com/techsupport.

Wiley also publishes its books in a variety of electronic formats. Some content that appears in print may not be available in electronic books.

British Library Cataloguing in Publication Data: A catalogue record for this book is available from the British Library

ISBN: 978-0-470-97449-0 (paperback), 978-0-470-97541-1 (ebk), 978-0-470-97542-8 (ebk), 978-0-470-97630-2 (ebk)

Printed and bound in Great Britain by TJ International, Padstow, Cornwall

10  9  8  7  6  5  4  3  2

WILEY

# About the Authors

**Tracy Packiam Alloway, PhD,** is the Director of the Center for Memory and Learning in the Lifespan at the University of Stirling, UK. She was the 2009 winner of the prestigious Joseph Lister Award by the British Science Association for bringing her scientific discoveries to a wide audience. She is the author of over 75 scientific articles and books on working memory and learning, and has developed the world's first standardised working-memory tests for educators, published by Pearson Assessment. Her research has received widespread international coverage, appearing in outlets such as the Scientific American, Forbes, US News, ABC News, BC, BBC, Guardian, and Daily Mail. She is a much-in-demand international speaker in North America, Europe, Asia, and Australia, and provides advice to the World Bank on the importance of working memory.

**Timothy E. Parker** is the Senior Crossword Puzzle Editor of *USA Today Crosswords* and the 'World's Most Syndicated Puzzle Compiler' according to *Guinness World Records*. In addition, he is the creator and senior editor of the *Universal Crossword,* the Internet's most popular crossword puzzle since 1998.

# Dedication

To Marcus: For teaching me that you are never too young to train your brain.

To Baby No. 2: For keeping me company while I was writing this book.

– Tracy Packiam Alloway, PhD

# Publisher's Acknowledgements

We're proud of this book; please send us your comments through our Dummies online registration form located at www.dummies.com/register/.

Some of the people who helped bring this book to market include the following:

**Commissioning, Editorial, and Media Development**

**Project Editor:** Steve Edwards

**Commissioning Editor:** Nicole Hermitage

**Assistant Editor:** Ben Kemble

**Development Editor:** Kelly Ewing

**Copy Editor:** Charlie Wilson

**Technical Editor:** Liam Healy

**Proofreader:** Anne O'Rorke

**Production Manager:** Daniel Mersey

**Cover Photos:**
© Mike Kemp/Rubberball/Corbis

**Cartoons:** Rich Tennant
(www.the5thwave.com)

**Composition Services**

**Project Coordinator:** Lynsey Stanford

**Layout and Graphics:**
Samantha K. Cherolis, Cheryl Grubbs

**Proofreader:** Lauren Mandelbaum

**Indexer:** Claudia Bourbeau

**Special Help**

**Brand Reviewer:** Carrie Burchfield

**Publishing and Editorial for Consumer Dummies**

**Diane Graves Steele,** Vice President and Publisher, Consumer Dummies

**Kristin Ferguson-Wagstaffe,** Product Development Director, Consumer Dummies

**Ensley Eikenburg,** Associate Publisher, Travel

**Kelly Regan,** Editorial Director, Travel

**Publishing for Technology Dummies**

**Andy Cummings,** Vice President and Publisher, Dummies Technology/General User

**Composition Services**

**Debbie Stailey,** Director of Composition Services

# Contents at a Glance

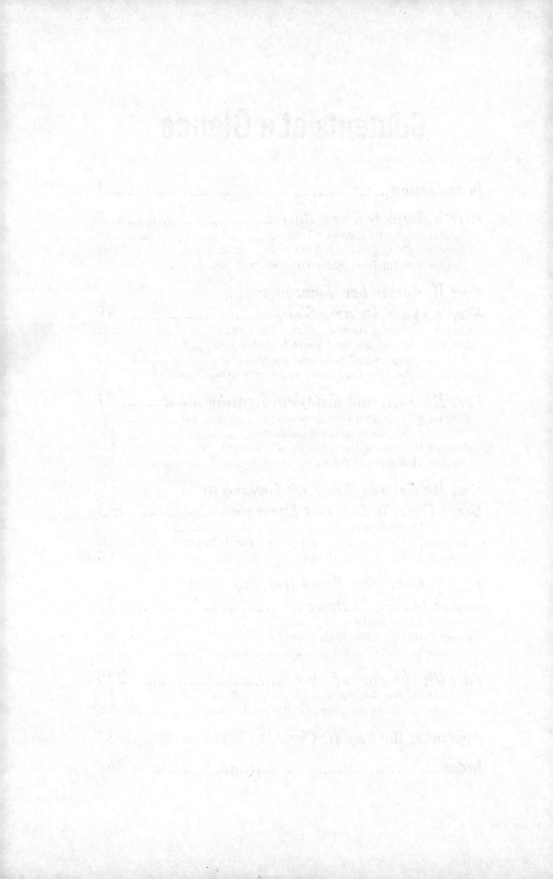

# Table of Contents

# Introduction

●　●　●　●　●　●　●　●　●　●　●　●　●　●　●　●　●　●　●　●　●　●　●　●　●　●　●　●　●　●　●　●　●　●　●　●　●　●　●　●　●　●

*1* imagine that you've picked up this book because you're interested in finding out more about the brain. In particular, I expect you're interested in what *you* can do to help your brain work better than it does now. Knowledge about the brain and how to train your brain has snowballed in recent years and keeping up with all the scientific research that's coming out is hard.

## About This Book

In this book I distil information into bite-sized chunks. I discuss a range of topics relevant to brain training, from computer games to what you should eat, even to what exercise is best for your brain, calling on cutting-edge science. In some of the topics I draw from my own research expertise, and in other topics I follow leading psychologists, scientists, and researchers in the field.

Each chapter deals with a different aspect of brain training, so by the time you get to the end of the book you have a complete picture of what you can do to boost your brain power. The strategies are simple, effective, and easy to fit into your busy lifestyle. You don't have to make major changes to make a big difference. Many of the tips and advice involve small changes that revolutionise your brain.

## Conventions Used in This Book

This book follows similar conventions to those that you may have come across in the *For Dummies* series. Here are some of the conventions that you see in the chapters:

- ✔ *Italics.* Words in italics are new words or keywords I introduce that are relevant to the chapter or the section. I always provide definitions for these keywords.

- ✔ **Sidebars.** I include interesting stories that are relevant to the chapter in the grey, shaded boxes. You don't have to read the sidebars, but I think they provide a nice way to see brain training tips in action.

# What You're Not to Read

If you've read a *For Dummies* book before, then you may be familiar with its characteristic relaxed style. You don't have to read this book from cover to cover to know what's going on. In fact, don't do that! Start with a section that you're interested in, and read that. Feel free to dip in and out of the chapters. As with all *For Dummies* books, the chapters are stand-alone so you can easily follow them without having to read the previous chapters.

# Foolish Assumptions

In writing this book, I've assumed that you want to know the essentials about how the brain works, and that you want to know what you can do in your daily life to help your brain work more efficiently.

To help fulfil these needs, I've included some cutting-edge scientific research on the brain as well, but not so much that things get boring! Whenever I mention psychologists or studies, I'm referring to actual published research. I've also included some stories from real-life situations that I hope you enjoy as well.

# How This Book Is Organised

This book has six parts. I provide you with tips, advice, strategies, and the science behind the ideas. Here's a breakdown of what you can expect.

## Part 1: Brain Training Basics

This part provides you with a step-by-step guideline to how the brain works and who the key players are. I also talk about common misconceptions about the brain, as well as frequently asked questions about brain training. The brain training software industry has exploded in the last few years, and I review a range of products for all ages. Find out the science behind these different programs (such as Nintendo's Brain Age) and discover whether they'll work to train your brain.

# Part II: Remember, Remember . . . Keeping Your Memory Sharp

From forgetting car keys to shopping lists, faces, and directions, everyone's experienced that feeling of 'what was it that I needed to do?'. In this part I talk about the different memory systems and what you can do to make your memory work better. Get tips to improve your verbal memory (language), visual memory (faces), and spatial memory (directions). So at the next company party, you'll be the only one who doesn't get lost on the way and remembers everyone's face and name!

# Part III: Fostering a Happy, Healthy Mind

Stress, anxiety, and depression can all take a toll on how your brain works. They can start to have a negative impact on your job, your relationships, and even your plans for the future. But it doesn't have to be this way. You can do many scientifically proven things to boost your mental health. Find out how to combat stress and anxiety and make happiness a daily choice. It really does make your brain work better. Probably one of the most fun ways to train your brain is to foster healthy friendships. Even digital friendships (through social networking) make a positive difference!

# Part IV: Getting Physical: Looking at Brain-Friendly Diet and Lifestyle

Brain-boosting food doesn't have to be boring – in this part you find out many delicious foods that you can eat and drink to improve your brain. I provide tips from pre-birth (pregnancy) to adulthood, so you have no excuse for not benefiting from what you're eating, no matter what your age. Also in this part is advice on what physical activities work best to enhance your brain's functioning.

# Part V: Game On! Brain Training Games to Play at Home

Ready to get started? Part V includes many different games that you can play to train your brain at home. Take your pick from language games, number games, and memory games.

# Part VI: The Part of Tens

The Part of Tens gives you top ten things that you can do to train your brain. In Chapter 18 you discover ten new things that you can do to make your brain more efficient. The tips are fun and enjoyable activities that everyone can (and should!) do.

Don't let the excuse of not having enough time stop you from training your brain. In Chapter 19 I give you ten things you can do to train your brain on the move.

# Icons Used in This Book

Icons are commonly used throughout *For Dummies* books and this one is no exception. Here's what each icon means.

This icon provides an anecdote, a study or an interesting fact that relates to the topic.

Don't skip this section – it's jam-packed with advice and strategies that you can begin using right away.

Doing some late night reading and only want one thing to take away? Then read this icon to find out more.

This icon provides a caution – whether it's what to avoid or what to be aware of; make sure you don't miss this.

Sometimes, a little pearl of wisdom is important to remember. This icon helps you to file away information that may help you to train your brain when the opportunity arises.

This icon relates to fairly in-depth information. You may want to flick past these paragraphs or stay there and find out more. When you can apply the information to training your brain, you may find the information here encouraging you to delve a little deeper into the subject.

# *Where to Go from Here*

Now what? Well, if you want change, it's now within your grasp. Start with a topic that you're interested in and dive in. But remember, reading this book alone won't increase your brain's efficiency. You must actually practise the strategies to see improvements. The first step to change is desire – do you want to change? By picking up this book you've already demonstrated that you do. The rest is easy.

# Part I
# Brain Training Basics

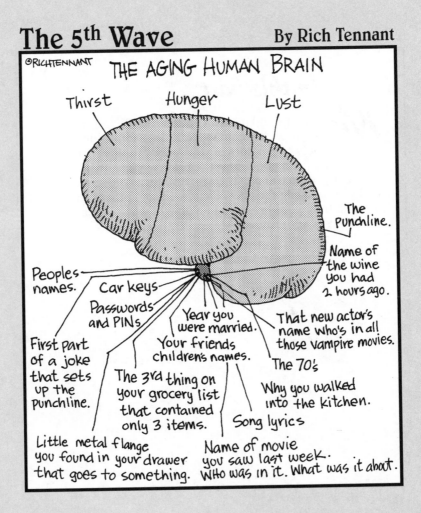

# In this part...

**M**any myths and misconceptions are floating around about how the brain works. For example, do you really use only 10 per cent of your brain? In this part you find out the truth about how the brain works and how you can easily begin training it. Brain training is one area that's really cutting-edge science. Clear evidence proves that you *can* train your brain, and I highlight what works best for different age groups.

# Chapter 1

# Introducing Brain Training

*E*veryone wants their brain to work at its best – whether you want to stay sharp to keep up with your children or come up on top at work. The exciting thing is that science now provides evidence for what works and what doesn't. So training your brain no longer has to be a case of trial and error – trying one thing, finding out that it doesn't work and then trying something else.

In this chapter I talk about cutting-edge, scientific research and examine how this research can influence your life and change your brain for the better.

## Yes, You Can Train Your Brain!

People who use their brain more efficiently tend to have better jobs, better relationships, and more happy and fulfilling lives. And here's the exciting thing: you can change your brain and, as a result, change your circumstances. Although you may have long been told that you're stuck with the brain you have, scientific research has now found that this isn't true!

*Brain plasticity* – the brain's amazing ability to adapt and change throughout your life – is an exciting and growing area. And the great thing is, you have the power to change your brain to help it function more effectively.

Brain training doesn't have to include a major overhaul of your life. Here are some straightforward tips to get you started:

 ✔ **No time?** Grab a handful of blueberries on your way out the door (Chapter 12); play a brain game while you're on the move (Chapter 19); and spend a few minutes each day in (Chapter 10).

 ✔ **No energy?** Find out the best exercise to boost your brain (your body will also thank you; Chapter 14); reap the benefits of green tea (Chapter 13); and discover the power of sleep for your brain (Chapter 14).

 ✔ **No motivation?** Friendships not only increase motivation, but they also improve your brain power! Spend just ten minutes socialising to experience the same benefits to your brain as doing a crossword puzzle (Chapter 11).

# Getting to Know Your Brain

You've heard of the left brain and the right brain. Well, it's true that the brain is made up of the left and right hemispheres and that they have different functions. However, it's not entirely true that some people are only 'left-brainers' and others are 'right-brainers'. For example, language skills are located in the left hemisphere (see Chapter 2) and everyone uses this part of the brain! You don't need to hide behind the excuse that you're a right-brainer so you can't remember names. With the activities included in this book, you can get both halves of your brain working at their optimum levels.

In the world of brain training, key players exist and I talk about how to keep them alert and active in Chapter 2. The most important thing to remember is that the different parts of the brain don't work in isolation – they come together like a team. When you train one part of the brain, the rest also benefits. You can think of the brain like an orchestra or like a sports teams. The message is the same – one star player can't carry the rest of the team. They all have to work together.

# The Long and Short of Memory

Your brain stores information that you come across briefly in your *short-term memory*. If you rehearse the information often, you can move it to your *long-term memory*. After the information is in your long-term memory, you usually have access to it indefinitely.

# The long story

Long-term memory is made up of many different types of memories:

- **Autobiographical memories.** Childhood memories and meaningful events, for example, are known as *autobiographical memories*. These types of memories are really powerful and the loss of them can be a good early indicator of dementia and Alzheimer's disease. You can do many things to keep these memories fresh; I discuss how in Chapter 4.

- **Semantic memory.** Your knowledge of facts and random bits of information is known as *semantic memory*, which is very useful in converting new information from your short-term memory into your long-term memory. Find what strategies for doing this work best in Chapter 4.

- **Procedural memory.** *Procedural memory* is an automatic skill that you don't even have to think about – like driving a car or writing your name. You can discover how to make new things become automatic in order to help your brain work more efficiently.

# The short story

Short-term memory is responsible for you remembering verbal, visual and spatial information. People don't usually remember things in their short-term memory for very long unless they make a conscious effort to 'move' them into long-term memory stores.

Here are a few different ways in which you use your short-term memory.

- **Verbal.** Do you forget what you were saying in the middle of a conversation? Find yourself standing on the top of the stairs and can't remember why you walked up there? These are common phenomena and aren't signs of serious of memory loss. However, if you want to keep your brain in top shape, find out how to keep your language skills sharp. Whether you want to remember your list of errands or avoid memory loss as you get older, keeping your brain active can overcome signs of Alzheimer's disease (see Chapter 6).

- **Visual.** Why do some people look so familiar, yet you struggle to remember their names? This is an example of visual memory at work. Use tricks to boost your brain when it comes to remembering faces and other types of visual information (see Chapter 7).

✔ **Spatial.** Do you always find yourself struggling to remember directions? Spatial memory holds the key to getting you to the right destination instead of ending up in the wrong neighbourhood. One trick is to adopt a bird's eye perspective when you're in a new place. Read Chapter 7 for more tips on how to improve your spatial memory skills.

# Developing a Healthy Brain

*Mental health* refers to your state of being. Are you happy? When do you find yourself frustrated? Do you feel stressed out? What makes you feel anxious? These questions are important in determining how well your brain functions. So make sure that you pay attention to your mental health – doing so can make the difference between living a fulfilled life and a frustrated one.

Don't take your passions and hobbies for granted. Discover how these can make your brain more creative. And a more creative brain is a smarter brain. Whether you're a music lover or a budding writer, you can choose from a range of activities to help your brain.

You can choose to be optimistic to make a difference to your mental health. You can easily think that a change in circumstances will change everything for you and make your life better. But this is seldom the case. The cautionary tale of the lottery winner in Chapter 9 demonstrates that – despite winning millions – he ended up unhappy and wishing he'd never even won in the first place! So how do you make yourself smile? Chapter 9 gives you a lot of ideas that you can easily try out.

Getting swept away in a myriad of things that demand your attention on a daily basis is easy. Yet in this ever-demanding environment, finding time to quiet your brain and create a space for contemplation is increasingly important. Calm time brings tremendous benefits for your brain. You don't have to be a nun or a monk and spend hours each time to experience the benefits of contemplation. Scientific research has found that even ten minutes a day makes a big difference in improving how your brain works. Read Chapter 10 to find out more and pick up pointers on what you can do in your daily life to make time for quiet.

One great way to train your brain is to keep it socially active. From picking up the phone, to meeting for coffee, to discussing the latest movie together – growing research illustrates the benefits of friendships for the brain.

And it's not just face-to-face interactions that make a positive impact. Virtual friendships can also boost your brain power! Digital technology is advancing, but be aware that not all digital technology benefits your brain. Only when you're actively engaging with digital technology can you also experience benefits to your cognitive skills. Read Chapter 11 for more advice.

# Getting Active for Life

An active lifestyle leads to a more efficient brain – one that can respond better to stress, remember information, and be more attentive. From what you eat, to what exercise you do, to how much sleep you get and the amount of caffeine you drink – all these affect your brain. Understanding how your daily decisions in these areas could be making a big difference to how your brain works is important. So before you take another bite of your sandwich or drink another glass of wine, find out what really is best for your brain.

Here is a quick overview of tips and strategies you can find in this book:

- ✔ **Eat for your brain.** Chocolate to boost your brain? Juice to help your memory? Steak to help your attention? Eating the right brain food doesn't mean that you end up eating lettuce and flavourless food. On the contrary, many delicious and wonderful foods are packed with nutrients that are fantastic for your brain. Read Chapter 12 before you start cooking so that you can eat the best foods for your brain.

- ✔ **Get help from stimulants.** Caffeine, alcohol, and medication – they're all a double-edged sword. In some instances stimulants can help your brain work better. But many of these stimulants come at a price. Not all stimulants are equal – and you could end up harming instead of helping your brain. Read Chapter 13 to make sure that you know what you're getting into before it's too late.

- ✔ **You've got to move it!** If you think that Chapter 14, which is all about exercise, is going to make you feel guilty for not getting a gym membership, don't worry. It won't. Instead, you find out how even the brain responds to physical activity, how you can keep depression and memory loss at bay, and even how to help your body heal faster. Chapter 14 is also about rest – the importance of sleep to ensure that your brain is in great working shape.

# Chapter 2

# Getting to Know Your Brain

*In This Chapter*

▶ Acquiring an inside look at your brain lobes

▶ Getting to know your left and right hemispheres

▶ Challenging brain myths: fact from fiction

*T*he brain weighs a mere 3 pounds, yet it's responsible for the smooth running of your whole body. With 100 billion cells, your brain is like a CEO of a giant corporation.

If you're wondering how something so small has so much responsibility, you're in the right place to find out. In this chapter I provide basic information on how your brain works. This understanding provides the foundation to knowing how to best train your brain.

## Discovering How the Brain Works

Understanding of the brain has come a long way since the notion of the four humours – black bile, yellow bile, phlegm, and blood. According to the ancient Greeks and Romans, an imbalance in one of these humours would result in illness and affect both mental and physical health. This dominant view remained firmly in place until the 19th century when modern medical research came on the scene.

Since then, scientists have made great strides in understanding how the brain works and each day brings exciting new discoveries. In current understanding you can divide the brain into four parts.

### The four-part brain

When Phineas Gage went to work on the morning of 13 September 1848, the 25-year-old probably had no idea that he was going to be immortalised in medical and psychology history for years to come.

Phineas was a railroad worker who suffered severe head injuries as the result of a blast – a long iron rod was lodged in his head, passing from the top of his head and exiting from his cheek (see Figure 2-1). Remarkably, Phineas survived! He could walk, communicate with his family and friends, and seemed aware of his surroundings. However, his personality changed completely, and he had great difficulty controlling his anger. He'd transformed from a mild-mannered young man to a violent and hot-tempered individual. People who knew him before his accident said that he was no longer the same Gage they knew.

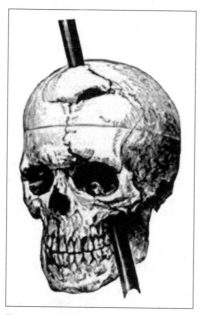

**Figure 2-1:** The skull of Phineas Gage with an image of the iron rod.

Phineas's injury provided the medical and psychology profession with great insight into how the brain works. By looking at the trajectory of the iron rod through his head, they were able to understand the link between different parts of the brain and everyday functioning.

Parts of the frontal lobe are linked to personality. Unfortunately for Phineas, this part of his brain sustained the most damage, which resulted in his dramatic change in character. Other sections of the frontal lobe are associated with language and motor skills, which, thankfully for Phineas, remained intact.

The four major areas of the brain are as follows (Figure 2-2 shows you where they're located):

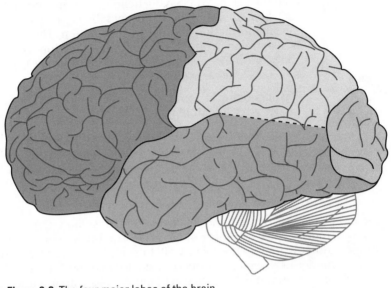

**Figure 2-2:** The four major lobes of the brain.

✔ **Frontal lobe.** As the name suggests, the frontal lobe is located in the front of the brain and makes up the largest part of the brain. One main function of the frontal lobe is to plan and organise incoming information. For example, if you have to plan a party, draw up the guest list and organise the catering, your frontal lobe is critical in carrying out all these activities.

The frontal lobe is also instrumental in regulating behaviour and emotions. This part of the brain, which is associated with a chemical known as *dopamine*, is sometimes called the brain's pleasure centre because it's linked to reward and enjoyment.

The frontal lobe doesn't fully develop until people reach their 20s, which may explain why it's so hard to convince a toddler to stop throwing a tantrum, or a teenager to consider the long-term consequences of her decisions. Both these scenarios involve the use of the frontal lobe to plan actions, consider consequences, and then alter actions as necessary.

✔ **Parietal lobe.** The parietal lobe is crucial in integrating information from a range of different sources, including sensory and visual information. The parietal lobe is divided into the right and left hemispheres (see the section on 'Looking at the Brain's Two Sides' in this chapter for more information).

✔ **Temporal lobe.** The temporal lobe is the home of language processing – Broca's area is located in this part of the brain (see the section on 'Saying hello to the left side' in this chapter). Some parts of the temporal lobe are responsible for visual information and object recognition. The temporal lobe is also home to another key player – the hippocampus (see the section 'Keeping the brain alert and active'), which is linked to long-term memory.

Throughout this book, I refer to the hippocampus and its role in everyday functioning (see Chapter 7 for an example).

✔ **Occipital lobe.** The occipital lobe is the smallest of the four lobes and is located at the back of the brain. It's home to the visual cortex and is responsible for processing visual information, perceiving motion, and detecting colour differences I don't discuss this part of the brain much in this book.

The parts of the brain don't function in isolation; they work together like members of an orchestra. But sometimes all the parts don't work together very well. In some cases, certain parts are under-performing but other parts are over-performing. One example of what this looks like is in individuals with attention-deficit hyperactivity disorder (ADHD). Research on ADHD has established that these individuals have underactive components in parts of their frontal lobe (responsible for planning and controlling behaviour) and an overactive motor cortex (necessary for managing motor functions). The combination of under-performance in one area and over-performance in another area results in the hyperactive and impulsive behaviour that's characteristic of ADHD.

## Keeping the brain alert and active

The *prefrontal cortex* is one of the most crucial parts of the brain. It's linked with *executive function* skills, which you use for everyday tasks like decision-making and planning.

For example, say you're driving down a busy road but you're late for a meeting. The bus-only lane is moving a lot faster, but you're not supposed to be in that lane. Should you go anyway? If you do, then you'll get to your meeting on time. You look at the queue and see that the police are ahead. You think that you've enough time to get in the bus lane and then get out before you reach the police car. This decision is an executive function skill.

Here's another scenario: the phone rings and it's someone giving you important information about an event that you're attending. You're busy writing all this information down when you hear a beep from your computer alerting you that an email has just come in from your friend. You run over and check your email, but as you're skimming it you get distracted and miss some of the information about the event.

# A lesson from the past: Lobotomising the prefrontal cortex

Your knowledge of a lobotomy may be based on Jack Nicolson's excellent portrayal of a rebellious patient at a mental hospital in the film *One Flew Over the Cuckoo's Nest*. According to the other patients in the hospital, a lobotomy effectively reduced someone to the same mental state as a shop window mannequin – expressionless and unemotional.

The lobotomy procedure consists of cutting the brain connections that go in and out of the prefrontal cortex (see 'Keeping the brain alert and active' for information on the prefrontal cortex). Doctors considered a lobotomy the final step for modifying extreme behaviour when other treatments, such as shock therapy or electrical shock treatment, failed to change a patient's behaviour. Doctors thought that a lobotomy calmed the patient, reduced aggressive behaviour, and improved the patient's quality of life. However, scientists now know that this procedure is no longer necessary.

Perhaps one of the youngest known recipients of a lobotomy is Howard Dully, who was only 12 years old at the time. As a result of a diagnosis of childhood schizophrenia (that was unconfirmed by other medical professionals at the time), Howard underwent the procedure. His mental illness manifested itself in some ways as a typical teenager – he was moody, insolent, and contrary. However, the truth behind his behaviour was harder to decipher – what was Dully really like and was his behaviour so extreme that a lobotomy was the only option? These questions have spawned Dully's lifelong search for answers.

He took several decades to recover, drifting from a mental institute, to prison, and finally to the streets. He's since overcome his setbacks and recounted his story in a harrowing tale of survival and redemption from a brutal procedure once considered acceptable by doctors but, thankfully, no longer in practice today.

Dully's story is interesting because it reveals that our knowledge of the brain is evolving. His journey has also served to fuel many heated discussions about how the brain works and the impact of removing sections of the brain.

Both these examples illustrate how you use your prefrontal cortex to make decisions that you're faced with daily. You have to keep a goal in mind (reaching your destination or writing down key information), juggle different scenarios (should you go in the carpool lane) or tasks (should you check your email while on the phone) and inhibit potentially distracting information to reach your goal (putting the thought of using the carpool lane out of your head; delaying the desire to read your email at that moment).

In addition to the prefrontal cortex, the hippocampus and amygdale are also key players in keeping your brain active and alert.

TRY THIS

Try This

# Testing your prefrontal cortex's function

Here's an example of a test to measure how well your prefrontal cortex works.

Say these words as fast as you can:

*Cat Dog Dog Cat Dog Cat Cat Dog Cat Dog*

Now say it when you see the pictures

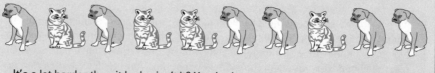

Now here's the tricky part: say the opposite word of what you see. If the word is *Cat*, say 'Dog'; if the word is *Dog*, say 'Cat'.

*Cat Dog Dog Cat Dog Cat Cat Dog Cat Dog*

How did you do? Here's a final one: say the opposite word of the picture.

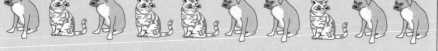

It's a lot harder than it looks, isn't it? You had to suppress or inhibit your automatic response to say the word rather than its opposite. You may be familiar with a more common version (called the *Stroop test*) where you have to state the colour that a word is printed in, rather than the actual word itself – for example the word 'blue' written in green ink.

### *Hippocampus*

The name *hippocampus* comes from the Greek word for seahorse, and it's called such because it looks very much like a seahorse. The hippocampus is in both the left and right sides of the brain. (For more on each side of the brain, see the section 'Looking at the Brain's Two Sides', later in this chapter.)

The hippocampus has two main functions: long-term memory and spatial understanding (see Chapter 4 for more information on long-term memory). The brain stores two types of long-term memories in the hippocampus:

✔ *Autobiographical memory* refers to meaningful events – birthdays, weddings, graduations and so on.

✔ *Declarative memory* is knowledge about facts, what you know about different things. The hippocampus also functions like a spatial map that helps with directions and navigation (see Chapter 7). So if you get lost often while you're driving, blame your hippocampus!

Damage to the hippocampus can result from Alzheimer's disease, oxygen deprivation and epilepsy that affects the temporal lobe, where the hippocampus is located. People who sustain damage to the hippocampus experience difficulties in forming new memories, a condition known as *anterograde amnesia*. This damage can also erode older memories (known as *retrograde amnesia*). However, if your hippocampus is damaged you still retain *procedural memory* – the ability to learn new motor tasks (see Chapter 4 for more on this topic). The fact that long-term memories are stored in different parts of the brain can explain why an amnesic patient may not be able to remember important events from her life, but may still be able to learn to play the guitar.

The hippocampus is also linked to mental health. Research into patients with depression has found that the hippocampus is usually smaller (by around 10 per cent) compared with those not suffering from depression. The actual reduction of the hippocampus depends on the frequency of depressive episodes, as well as the length of time the depression went untreated. The result of a smaller hippocampus is that depression sufferers are unable to absorb new information (*declarative memory*). A number of antidepressants target these impairments associated with the reduction in the hippocampus (see Chapter 9 for tips to boost your mental health).

### Amygdala

The name *amygdala* comes from the Greek word for almond, due to its physical similarity to that nut. The amygdala is associated with emotional memories – those that make you laugh and those that make you cry.

The amygdala also helps you store information over the long term. If you have an emotional connection to the information you're trying to learn, you're more likely to transfer this knowledge to your long-term memory. For example, if you're trying to learn a new language, associate the new words with an emotional memory to help you make those words stick.

The amygdala is also linked with higher creative activity (see Chapter 8 for more on boosting your creative skills).

---

## Lateralised brain

The term *lateralised* refers to the idea that certain functions of the brain are more dominant in one hemisphere than another. One clear example of this is in the dominant hand – right- or left-handedness. But the idea of being a 'left-brained' or a 'right-brained' person is a misconception. Take the example of handedness. Although the majority of right-handed people have left-brain dominance for language, a much smaller proportion of left-handed people have right-brain dominance for language. In truth, the notion of the lateralised brain can vary between people as well as different brain functions. Although clear strengths are associated with each hemisphere of the brain, people often apply the concept of brain lateralisation to other areas, such as business management, which has no scientific basis.

---

# Looking at the Brain's Two Sides

Most people are aware that the brain is divided into the left hemisphere and the right hemisphere and is connected by a 'bridge' called the *corpus callosum*. But did you know that each hemisphere of the brain has different functions?

## Saying hello to the left side

Language is the most common function associated with the left hemisphere. Grammar, vocabulary and reading are all linked with the left hemisphere (see Chapter 6 for tips on how to improve your language skills).

The left hemisphere is associated with language skills (see the nearby sidebar 'Broken speech in Broca'). Brain imaging studies have found that typical readers use the left occipital temporal region, known as the *word forming area*, to sound out words while reading. Does the dyslexic brain also reveal this same pattern? A recent study looked at a group of 20-year-olds who'd been diagnosed with dyslexia in kindergarten. Brain imaging scans found very little activation in the left temporal area; instead the 20-year-olds had greater activation in the right temporal area. Some psychologists suggest that dyslexic students bypass mental pathways in the left brain areas associated with phonological awareness skills and rely instead on more visual methods to support their reading.

# Broken speech in Broca

We have Paul Broca to thank for furthering understanding about the language centre in the brain. It was his first patient who led him to this discovery. The patient could only speak the word *tan*, which Broca discovered was caused by damage to the brain tissue in the left hemisphere. He subsequently realised that this part of the brain was critical for speech production and affected other patients with similar brain damage. The part of the brain associated with language is now known as *Broca's area*.

Today, damage in Broca's area can be characterised by not only difficulty in language production but also in language comprehension. Such patients have a difficult time understanding the meaning of sentences. An example of an ambiguous sentence is 'The horse raced past the barn fell'. Such sentences are known as *garden path sentences* because although they're grammatically correct, they lead the reader down the path to incorrectly interpret the meaning of the sentence. These sentences are especially tricky for those with damage in Broca's area.

## *Getting to know the right side*

The right hemisphere controls actions on the left side of the body. It's responsible for spatial skills and recognising faces (see Chapter 7), as well as other visual processing. The right hemisphere also controls the thinking skills. Damage to this area can lead to difficulties in reasoning, attention problems, and even poor memory for visual images.

Researchers have used split brain experiments to understand more about how the right and left hemispheres work together. As a treatment for epilepsy, the corpus callosum (the bridge that links the two hemispheres) is cut. This prevents information from crossing between the two hemispheres.

Here's how a typical experiment works. A picture of a dog flashes up on the right side of a computer screen and, therefore, of the visual field. Because this image is processed by the left hemisphere, which deals with language, the patient is easily able to recognise the picture and says 'Dog'. However, if the picture flashes up on the left side of the computer side (processed by the right hemisphere), the patient says she can't see anything! Without the corpus callosum intact to link information between the two hemispheres, the right hemisphere of the brain is unable to communicate to the left hemisphere what it sees, and therefore the person can't translate what she sees into language.

## Aliens exist

Contrary to the name, *alien hand syndrome* isn't the latest sci-fi movie offering or a book on UFOs. This syndrome usually occurs in patients who've had the left and right hemispheres of the brain separated through a stroke or brain injury, or in severe cases of epilepsy. Patients who have alien hand syndrome can feel normal sensations, such as pain, cold and heat, in their hand. However, they feel that their hand isn't in their control and has a mind of its own. One example is where one hand buttons a shirt while the other immediately unbuttons it seemingly without being under the conscious control of the person. A woman in her 30s described how she would sit on her left hand when reading a book because it kept turning back the pages she turned with her right hand!

Amputees also experience this syndrome where they complain of pain or itching in their missing limb. Neuroscientist Dr Ramachandran has developed a way to help these patients by remapping the brain using optical illusions. He puts a mirror in a cardboard box and asks the patient to put her existing hand in the box next to the mirror. He then asks the patient to imagine that the image of the hand reflected in the mirror is her missing hand. The patient clenches and unclenches her fist while looking in the mirror. After a few weeks the patient reports that her pain in her missing arm has disappeared. According the Dr Ramachandran, this simple procedure using a mirror remaps the brain to align it with the reality of what the body is experiencing.

# Separating Fact from Fiction

They're like urban myths – 'facts' about the brain. You heard it from a friend, who heard it from a neighbour, who heard it from her boss. But how many of these facts are really true? In this section I discuss three widespread brain 'facts'.

## Do you really only use 10 per cent of your brain?

No evidence supports this statement. Although this idea has been highly popular (see sidebar 'Bending the truth'), no research whatsoever demonstrates that people only use a small portion of their brain.

Here are a few examples of how you can be sure that this statement is fictional.

✔ **Look inside.** Brain imaging techniques clearly reveal that people use all their brains (see the section "Discovering how the brain works' in this chapter for more information). Although you may use only a small part of your brain for a simple activity, whenever you engage in a complex activity you're using several parts of your brain simultaneously. A useful analogy is to think of your muscles. When you're eating, you may only be using your muscles relevant for chewing and swallowing. But that doesn't mean that you only ever use 10 per cent of your muscle group. In fact, it sounds ludicrous just to suggest that! In the same way, you use all of your brain at one point or another in a single day.

✔ **Using the whole brain.** The idea of only using 10 per cent of the brain suggests that the brain has very specialised purposes – that you only need certain parts of the brain to function efficiently. The other 90 per cent of the brain is like tonsils or the appendix – it's there, but you don't really need it for anything important. This is *not* true. Even damage to a small area of the brain caused by a stroke, head injury or certain disorders like Parkinson's disease has a devastating impact on the brain. The damage caused by these conditions is far less than damage to 90 per cent of the brain and yet it can leave people with difficulty speaking, remembering loved ones and even forming new memories. All the brain is necessary to function successfully.

✔ **Say baaa.** The average human brain weighs about 3 pounds (1,400 grams). If you removed 90 per cent of the brain, this would only leave about 0.3 pounds of brain tissue (140 grams). This brain size is much the same as a sheep's brain. So, the next time someone tells you that people only use 10 per cent of the brain, say baa!

## Does your brain shrink as you get older?

The short answer is yes, but not as much as you think – and brain training can make a difference. As you get older your brain does shrink around 2 per cent every ten years. This shrinkage actually begins in early adulthood but is unlikely to be noticeable until you hit your 60s. A greater percentage of brain shrinkage is linked with dementia. In other words, a certain amount of brain shrinkage is normal, but too much is a tell-tale sign of problems like Alzheimer's and dementia.

# Bending the truth

The notion that people only use 10 per cent of the brain was made especially popular in the 1990s by psychics who wanted to promote the idea that if you only use a small portion of your brain then you can develop the rest of the brain for psychic activities. You may have heard of a psychic named Uri Geller whose claim to fame is his ability to bend spoons and make broken watches work again. How does he do it? In his writings Uri attributed his fantastical 'achievements' like spoon bending and telepathic ability to him harnessing the unused 90 per cent of his brain.

However, as is so often the case, the truth is much less fantastical. The spoon bending trick is thought to be the result of misdirecting the audience's attention to focus on something else and then revealing an existing bend. In fact, when Uri was asked to perform his signature trick on silverware that he didn't have access to, he failed. His famous clock-starting trick was thought to be the result of using magnets, as slow-motion television footage revealed. So if you were hoping to harness the so-called 'idle 90 per cent' of your brain for spoon-bending activities, you may want to start with plastic spoons.

To avoid or at least delay major brain shrinkage, pay attention to these tips:

✔ **Pass on the alcohol.** Studies confirm that alcohol isn't great for your brain. In addition to all the negative health side effects, it makes your brain smaller. Even light drinkers (and by 'light' I mean 1–7 alcoholic drinks per week) suffer these effects of alcohol on the brain. A study that looked at people in their 60s found that even light drinkers had a smaller brain volume compared with those who abstained from alcohol. Heavy drinkers – those who drank more than 14 drinks each week – suffered the most when it came to brain volume.

Take special care if you're a woman – the brain volume of women is more affected by alcohol than men, meaning that the effects of light drinking can be more pronounced in women compared to men.

Why does alcohol affect brain volume? Alcohol dehydrates your tissues, and when this happens constantly your most sensitive tissue – your brain – starts getting affected (see Chapter 13 for more on stimulants and the brain).

✔ **Relax.** Stress can also impact your brain (see Chapter 9 for more on developing a positive mindset and learning to relax). This happens especially when you experience repeated stress, such as a prolonged illness or difficulty at work.

The prefrontal cortex, linked to decision-making and attention, and the hippocampus, linked to long-term memory, are most affected by stress (see the earlier section 'Keeping the brain alert and active'). Stress makes it harder for people to focus on the task at hand or take in new information. When people are stressed they lose their ability to be mentally flexible. This means that even when they're confronted with familiar problems, they find it difficult to solve them in new and creative ways.

✔ **Teach yourself.** You now know that brain shrinkage is normal. But this shrinkage doesn't have to impact the way your brain works. In fact, studies have demonstrated that people in their 60s to 90s are able to 'buffer' the effects of brain shrinkage. How? Simple: they kept their brain active by learning new things. People who spend time discovering and learning something they didn't know give their brains more protection against dementia and memory loss. By keeping up your intellectual activity, you're mentally exercising your brain to keep it fit as you grow older. If you can't wait, flip to Chapter 18 to discover ten new ways to buffer your brain from the effects of aging.

## Can you change your brain?

Yes! Yes! Yes! The exciting news is that the effects of aging aren't permanent. You can do something to reverse the consequences of aging on your brain. The brain has a certain *plasticity*, which means that you can change. This whole book is dedicated to providing you with tips on what you can do to make a difference to your brain and see results.

Scientific evidence has shown that performing certain activities can change your brain. Here are a few examples:

✔ **Brain training.** The idea of brain training is a new and exciting area of research and growing evidence suggests that you can do something to change your brain. However, be aware that not all brain training products give you the same results. In Chapter 3, I discuss what works and what doesn't.

✔ **Move it.** Exercise isn't only good for your body, it's great for your brain too! Some people say that the brain is like a muscle so you should exercise it. Well, there *is* a plasticity to the brain, but exercise is more than just exercising a muscle. For starters, exercise increases the blood flow to your brain, which helps it work better. Physical activity can also renew parts of the brain that are damaged and lead to new brain stem cells. This means better memory and an improved ability to learn. Read Chapter 14 to find out what types of exercise make the biggest difference in boosting your brain power.

✔ **Make time for bingo.** If exercise sounds like too much work for you, you'll be happy to know that socialising is also great for your brain. Studies have found that when people spend time interacting, the brain releases a feel-good hormone – *oxytocin* – which can boost memory (see Chapter 11 for more on this topic).

# Chapter 3

# Brain Training for Your Needs

· · · · · · · · · · · · · · · · · · · · · · · · · · · · · · · · · · · · · · · · · ·

· · · · · · · · · · · · · · · · · · · · · · · · · · · · · · · · · · · · · · · · · · ·

*B*rain training is a growing area of interest both in research and in the public mind. Exciting emerging evidence indicates that you can train your brain, and, as a result, you can change your circumstances. But what works and what doesn't? And can everyone benefit from brain training? This chapter looks at these issues in more detail.

## Brain Training in Children

Brain training in children is a hot topic. Just imagine the possibilities if you could improve the way a child thinks! Certainly, that's the view that some scientists have taken in light of exciting research findings. Parents too are equally excited about the possibilities of developing their child's thinking and reasoning skills.

This section discusses the best brain training for a child.

### Providing a stimulating environment for the brain

With so many products on the market that claim to 'improve your child's brain', how can you know which to choose? Read this section to know fact from fiction when it comes to brain training for children.

When a product claims to train your child's brain, look for the magic three in the product's clinical trials: transfer effects, control group and randomised samples.

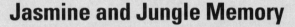

# Jasmine and Jungle Memory

Jasmine is a sweet 10-year-old whom I recently encountered. She wanted desperately to fit in with the other girls in her class. But the trouble was that Jasmine stood out, no matter how hard she tried. She stood out because she couldn't remember what the teacher said. She was the last in class to get ready for the lesson because she forgot what books she needed, and she was in the lowest ability group in literacy and maths. She knew that the other kids would laugh because she had a special assistant to help her in the classroom. Emma, Jasmine's mum, was also concerned about her. At home Jasmine would also get frustrated. Some evenings Emma found her daughter crying alone in her room because she couldn't remember what she was supposed to do. Simple tasks like tidying up and organising her books for school the next day seemed to overwhelm Jasmine.

You may be wondering why Jasmine struggled. In a recent assessment by the school psychologist she was identified at the bottom percentile in working memory. This is why she forgot the teacher's instructions and why she struggled in maths. Armed with this information, Emma looked for solutions and came across *Jungle Memory* in her search. Jasmine used the programme over the summer. When she started school in September her teacher was amazed. She said that Jasmine was a completely different student, and you wouldn't know that she had learning difficulties. Jasmine was no longer classified as a student with special learning needs; she no longer needed extra help in the classroom, and her grades improved. Emma noticed a big improvement at home as well. Jasmine could accomplish what she needed to do without feeling frustrated. When Jasmine was retested by the school psychologist her IQ had increased to the top 10 per cent for her age and her working memory had improved to an average level.

*Transfer effects* means asking this question: does the product improve anything other than getting better at the game itself? Of course, you'd expect that practising hard at one thing naturally makes you better at it. This is known as a *practice effect* – doing something enough times makes you good. But the real question is: can a brain training programme transfer to real world activities? In other words, can you get better at something other than the training game itself? That's the first question you need to ask yourself when you look at a brain training product.

Here's the second question: does a control group exist? A *control group* offers a comparison to make sure that the brain training programme isn't just working because the child is doing something different. Some studies just use a control group composed of people who don't do anything, but this doesn't offer a good comparison for the effectiveness of the training programme. An ideal control group is a group of people who are doing something different from the brain training programme (such as reading).

The final issue is whether the trials randomly assigned people to the training group or the control group: *randomised samples*. The trials shouldn't selectively assign people to a group.

When a clinical trial meets all these requirements, you can be assured that the results from the study are likely to be reliable. In other words, if the company offering a brain training product followed the magic three in its clinical trials and the results show that their product actually does improve skills, then the company's programme probably works.

Here are some tips for improving a child's brain power.

- ✔ **Turn off the computer games.** Some schools use specific computer games for this purpose. Although the games may be enjoyable, does any evidence exist to suggest they can improve learning? One study compared the benefits of playing certain computer games to playing Scrabble in school children. Can you guess which group performed the best on memory tests? It wasn't the computer game-playing group – it was the group that played Scrabble and word puzzles. So if you want your child to excel, it may be best to turn off the computer and buy a game of Scrabble instead.

- ✔ **Don't just memorise numbers.** Does memorising phone numbers improve the brain? Several brain training programmes use this approach. Students train in remembering a random sequence of numbers or locations daily for a few weeks. But sadly, although some students may get higher working memory scores after training, their grades don't actually improve immediately after training. Why? For the simple reason that these brain training programmes are just training for the test – if a child memorises numbers for a few weeks then of course he'll do better on a memory test of numbers. These improvements are known as a practice effect.

- ✔ **Try Jungle Memory.** In my own research I wanted to look at the transfer effects of brain training – can training a child's brain lead to better scores in learning? I looked at a programme called Jungle Memory (www.junglememory.com), which trains working memory together with key learning activities like reading and maths.

  I took a group of students with learning difficulties and randomly assigned them to one of two groups. Half of the students received brain training using Jungle Memory (training group), and the remaining students received targeted learning support in school (control group). I measured the students' IQs, working memory and learning scores before they started training. At the start of the trials both groups performed similarly on all these cognitive tests. This fact is important because it means that any improvements a child makes after training is the result of the training, rather than because he started at different level.

After training, the results were dramatic. The control group didn't perform any better. In contrast, the training group using Jungle Memory made great improvements in IQ, working memory, and most importantly, their learning scores. They increased their grades from a C to a B and from a B to an A in just eight weeks! This news is very exciting because improvements are immediately evident after training.

## Sesame Street versus Dr Seuss

When it comes to television, you may wonder just how harmful is that colourful screen? Can educational programmes help a child's brain?

In a study of over 2,000 children aged between 1 and 3 years old, psychologists found that for every hour of television a 1- to 3-year-old watched, these children had a 10 per cent greater chance of developing attention problems (such as ADHD) by the time they were 7 years old. Psychologists also found that a toddler watching three hours of baby videos every day had a 30 per cent higher chance of having attention problems in school.

Why? The changing images of the baby videos eventually over-stimulate a child, causing problems to his developing brain patterns. Even images that change at a slower pace cause problems to a child's brain development.

The consistent sounds of the television can also interfere with the child's development of their *inner voice* when they're learning to vocalise events. At this stage, children learn to develop their thought process, to think through things in order to respond appropriately. Having television on as a constant backdrop in his environment actually hinders a child from being able to develop his inner voice, which is critical for language development.

## Making the most of the early years

Scientists now know that the brain grows at an amazing rate during the first few years of life. In fact, a newborn's brain is only 25 per cent of its adult weight. By the age of 2 the baby's brain is 80 per cent of its adult weight.

TECHNICAL STUFF

# The Mozart Effect

You may have heard the phrase *Mozart effect,* which refers to the idea that listening to Mozart can actually improve your child's IQ. The idea came from an experiment conducted on a small group of college students who were asked to listen to a Mozart sonata. The psychologists found an improvement of spatial reasoning skills (see Chapter 7). But this improvement lasted for only ten minutes!

When a product makes claims that Mozart will make your child smarter, surely you hope that this improvement in IQ is going to last more than ten minutes! However, the original study clearly indicates that this effect doesn't last for any longer than this: it's temporary. And no, having your child listen to Mozart for a longer time won't increase his IQ for an extended period of time.

No reliable scientific studies show that listening to Mozart makes children any smarter, for any length of time. In fact, many studies have failed to replicate the so-called Mozart effect. One Harvard scientist examined the Mozart effect in 16 different studies with over 700 participants (that's almost 20 times more participants than in the original study, making the conclusions much more reliable). Yet none of these studies provided any scientific evidence for the Mozart effect. This is important to note, because when no one else is able to reproduce a scientific finding, the original findings are likely to have been a fluke. The premise that listening to Mozart will make your child smarter is simply false.

Your baby has almost all the nerve cells (neurons) at birth, and these nerve cells make important new connections after birth. These connections help the baby not only in the basic sensory skills such as sight, hearing, feeling and taste, but also in more complex skills such as thinking, acting and feeling. The rate at which these connections develop depends on external stimulation. This means that the more sensory stimulation babies have, the more connections their brain is able to form. For example, medical studies have found that children who aren't touched or don't play often develop brains 20 per cent to 30 per cent smaller than their peers.

This plasticity of the brain means that babies are extremely malleable and pick up environmental influences like a sponge. Particularly in the first two years of their lives, your baby is undergoing incredible changes in his mental development. This period is critical in helping your child grow mentally, socially and emotionally. Don't short-change your child by limiting his world to a 3 foot by 3 foot box.

Here are some suggestions of what you can do to develop your child's developing mental skills:

✔ **Sing to your child.** Your baby then develops a rhythm of communicating with you in music. You don't have to have a good voice. Your child just wants to hear you. Studies show that babies mimic the mother's voice and tone when she's talking to them. This path is an early stage to learning language and is very important in developing the rhythm of language.

✔ **Read aloud to your child.** Reading allows a child to engage in the images and colours and sounds in front of him while interacting with you. Reading is a powerful way to help a child connect words on the page with the sounds he makes. Reading is a great way to give your child a head start in life.

✔ **Talk about your world around you.** Remember that it's still a novelty for babies to see many things in a garden or while driving or going for a walk. Use this time to point out flowers, maybe a snail or a colourful butterfly. Take time to talk about the colours, how they're moving, why they're moving. All these things are new to your baby, and he's fascinated by his environment. You don't need to be an expert on the subject – just draw your child's attention to the physical features of an object, like the colour or the shape. You can say things like, 'Look at that snail. Its shell is round, just like your red ball.' This comparison helps your child make connections about the world around him.

✔ **Let your child try things out.** Children are naturally curious, so let your child see what happens when he mixes children's water paints and water, or maybe let him try touching a piece of dough or squishing a tomato between his fingers. You can even talk about mixing different paint colours to discover more about colour combinations. The important thing is to encourage your child, to encourage his curiosity and to let him explore the world around him (within safe boundaries!).

✔ **Make your child a part of your activities.** Whether you're cooking, washing dishes, making a phone call or shopping at the supermarket, let your child see what you're doing and take part in your activities when he can. If your child's old enough, make some cookies with him. Children learn from watching what you do, so encourage your child to copy your behaviour while you're cooking or cleaning. Your child will love participating, and you'll have precious memories to keep of your time together.

# Brain Training for Adults

As an adult, if you want to keep your brain active, you need to do something about it. The exciting news is that it's never too late to train your brain. At any age, you can see benefits for your brain.

## Dispelling the myths of brain training

With the increase of brain training, people throw around many 'facts'. The following list covers some of the more common statements about brain training:

- ✔ **You're stuck with what you have.** A long-held view is that you're born with what you have, and you can't do anything about it. For example, if you have a poor memory, then you'd better carry a notebook to help you remember! However, exciting developments in scientific research show that you can train your brain. The brain has a certain *plasticity* – this means that it can change (see Chapter 2 for more on brain plasticity). Studies show that at any age you can do something to make a difference.

- ✔ **Your brain age declines as you get older.** Here again, the general view is that things get worse as you get older. But recent evidence shows that this isn't the case. In fact, I looked at working memory in people from 5 to 85 years of age. Working memory skills continue developing in the 20s and peak in the 30s. And actually very little decline in working memory skills occurs. Working memory in people in their 60s looks like those in their 20s. So now you don't have an excuse for why you forgot to pick up milk on the way home!

- ✔ **All brain training is the same.** Unfortunately, this isn't the case. Many programmes claim to train your brain, but not all the programmes work. Evaluating each programme to decide whether evidence demonstrates that the programme is effective is important. Check to make sure that the magic three are evident in a programme's scientific trials (see the earlier section 'Providing a stimulating environment for the brain').

- ✔ **Only one way to train your brain exists.** As Chapter 2 highlights, the brain has four main lobes and many key areas involved in making your brain work like a smooth running machine. No single thing makes a difference. Each chapter in this book highlights a different strategy to keep your brain active, from what you eat to how much you sleep, to what to drink. Follow the tips to maximise your brain's potential.

## Using what works for your brain

Make sure that the brain training programmes that you use to train your brain have these key features:

✔ **Adaptive training.** *Adaptive training* means that the training programme changes to your needs and your ability. This means that you won't always work at the same level each time, but if you're doing well then the programme challenges you with harder levels, and if you're struggling, then the programme should move to an easier level. Adaptive training is important to continue to challenge your brain.

✔ **Speed up.** Studies have found that programmes that use timed tasks to train your brain to work faster make a difference. Practising timed tasks makes a difference to everyday activities as well. Even if you aren't using a computer-based training programme, try timing yourself when you solve a crossword or Sudoku. You'll notice yourself get faster and even banish that tip-of-the-tongue phenomenon (see Chapter 6 for more strategies).

✔ **Keep it regular.** Training regularly is important. If you only use a programme once a week, don't expect to see results. Studies have found that you need to train at least three times a week to see maximum benefits for your brain. So don't be lazy – and get training.

Tetris is an old favourite for many people. This game consists of rotating coloured blocks in such a way that you avoid reaching the top of the screen. With each level the speed increases to challenge the player. Now fans of Tetris can play with impunity – scientific evidence is on your side! Research shows that spatial memory improves after playing Tetris. Not only that, some scientists have also observed physical changes in the brain after playing Tetris for an extended period and that the brain worked more efficiently in some tasks. Not a bad result for just rotating some coloured blocks on the screen!

Goodbye puzzles? In a recent survey people reported that they preferred to use computerised products than puzzle books. This may explain why brain training products have skyrocketed in recent years. However, don't give up on puzzles and board games. Strong evidence indicates that these activities keep your brain active. Even schoolchildren benefit more from playing board games like Scrabble than playing on a computer game (see the earlier section 'Providing a stimulating environment for the brain'). So don't stop playing word games, doing crosswords or challenging your spouse to late-night Scrabble; it's great for your brain (see Chapters 15 to 17 for more ideas on brain training games).

# BBC study

Recently the BBC thought it would be a good idea to run a mass-participation brain training study. About 11,000 people volunteered to sign up for the online project and the BBC assigned each participant to one of three groups. In the first group – reasoning brain training – people had to solve tasks that involved planning and analysing the problem to come up with a response. They had to choose problems from categories like pop music and history. In the second group – non-reasoning brain training – people had tasks that involved short-term memory and attention tasks. And the final group – the control group – didn't actually participate in any training but spent a similar amount of time on the computer as the reasoning and non-reasoning brain training groups.

What were the results? The first finding was that people got better at the task – the *practice effect*. In other words, playing the reasoning games meant that people got better at those types of tasks. In contrast, the control group didn't show any improvement in reasoning tasks, which isn't surprising given that they weren't training at all.

The next finding was that none of the training transferred to any other tasks. So although people got better at the training games, that didn't help them perform better in other activities. Although this result may seem surprising, several reasons exist:

- ✔ The first is that the games themselves were targeting very specific knowledge-based activities, like history or pop music. So perhaps it's not that surprising that knowing a lot about pop music won't help you remember your shopping list.

- ✔ Another problem is that the group of people participating in the study was self-selecting, which means that the participants chose to sign up, and they weren't monitored by rigorous experimental procedure. Big differences in how regularly people chose to use the training programme existed, which may have affected the results.

- ✔ And an additional issue was that the participants were highly educated and aged between 18 and 60 years of age. The training programme may have been too easy for the participants, and as a result the programme may not have challenged the participants sufficiently to see any benefits of training.

So what's the bottom line? Brain training does work. You just need to make sure that you're doing the right thing.

# Part II
# Remember, Remember . . . Keeping Your Memory Sharp

## The 5th Wave

By Rich Tennant

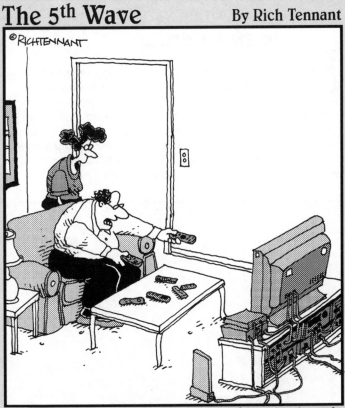

"I don't know why people say watching TV doesn't challenge your brain. You've got to be a genius to figure out which remote operates the TV, cable, Wii, volume, DVD player, channel, VCR..."

## *In this part...*

**I**s forgetting your keys all the time a sign of your brain getting older? Can't remember faces or phone numbers? Trouble finishing the end of your sentences? In this part I list tips and strategies to help you remember everything from directions, to faces, to phone numbers. I also talk about how short-term memory (remembering something for a short time) works together with long-term memory to keep your brain working at its best.

# Chapter 4

# Honing Your Long-Term Memory

*L*ong-term memory is when you retain information for a long period of time. You may remember some of this information, like a memorable birthday, for years and years, yet other memories don't last more than a week.

Think of long-term memory like a library full of books. Some books get read more than others so it's easier to remember which shelf you left them on. With long-term memory, some experiences are better remembered than others because you think about them more.

In Chapter 5, I discuss short-term memory, which is like the check-out table in the library. You keep a few books in front of you, but you don't always remember the information for a long period.

## Remembering Your Past: Autobiographical Memory

One of my favourite stories from my childhood is one my mother tells of when I was 3 years old. I was spending some time with my aunt and grandmother one afternoon. After exhausting all options for playing, I wandered into my grandmother's room and proceeded to throw her watch and precious jewellery out of the window. None of this might have been so bad, except that my aunt lived on the top floor of a very high apartment building. Needless to say, my grandmother's watch and jewellery came crashing down on the street to the surprise of the passers-by! None of the items survived the fall.

Do I remember any of this? Not at all. Yet your childhood memories can play an important role in keeping your brain alert. Why? For starters, remembering past experiences is important because they serve as a template for how to solve present and future problems. These types of memories act as a guide for both brain and behaviour in responding and reacting successfully when presented with a challenging situation. Past experiences, such as your childhood memories, also act like a bridge to connect new information with stored knowledge.

## *Discovering the importance of childhood memories*

It's often hard to remember memories before the age of 3 because language skills aren't well developed. If you can't speak, how can you talk about what you did that day? And if you can't articulate what you did, how can you add it to the library shelf of your long-term memory?

Another reason why memories from a very young age are hard to remember is because the brain is not fully developed then. In Chapter 7 I talk about the hippocampus. This part of the brain plays an important role in consolidating memories and it's not fully developed before two years of age. This makes it hard for very young children to form connections between their experiences and transfer that into their long-term memory library.

 To remind yourself of your happy childhood memories, take a walk down memory lane. Flick through your photo albums to trigger happy holidays, and read through old birthday cards and letters that you've exchanged with loved ones. Sometimes you can forget how many happy moments you've had and reminding yourself is important. Don't store your photo albums in a hard-to-reach place like an attic. Instead, keep albums in a prominent place like a bookshelf so you can reach for them regularly.

 Not all memories are reliable. A *false memory*, as the name suggests, is a memory of an event that never happened or an embellishment of an event that did happen. This occurrence is most common with childhood memories. You may remember an event that never occurred, such as owning a rabbit when you were little. You can also have a memory that elaborates on an event that did actually occur. If, for example, you had a dog as a pet, you may remember that you and your dog used to chase rabbits in the nearby field. However, your parents may point out that you lived in a busy city with no fields nearby.

# I know that you did it!

False memories can appear in adulthood. You may remember an incident with a friend that never actually occurred or a trip that you never took. Although most of these memories are usually quite harmless, sometimes they can cause a problem. Eyewitness testimony is one such example. People are actually very bad at remembering important details and are easily misled by the questions people ask. Psychologists tested this theory with a group of adults by showing video footage of a car accident. The psychologists asked one group to estimate the speed of the car when it *hit* another car. They asked the other group the same question, but using the phrase '*smashed* the other car'. People in the second group 'remembered' broken glass in the video footage although no broken glass was present at all! It seems that when you ask people a misleading question, their memory of the event is wrong.

Other studies have found that when something is shocking in an event, like a man holding a gun, people only focus on the gun and can't remember what the man looks like. Imagine what happens when an observer sees a crime. So much is going on – people are yelling, cars are honking, everything seems a little crazy. Can you really expect that memory of the criminal's face to be reliable? What if the man was wearing a hat or covering his face? How can witnesses be sure of what they saw?

It's actually quite difficult to recognise someone's face. One tip is to immediately focus on something distinctive like facial hair or piercings. This can make it a little easier to identify someone at the crime scene. You can also write down what you saw right away. Chapter 7 provides more suggestions on how to improve your memory for faces, whether for business, pleasure, or as a critical eyewitness to a crime.

## *Harnessing the power of happy memories*

Emotions play a big role in how much you remember. You may remember something from your childhood because you did it all the time, like spending all summer at the local swimming pool. Other memories last because they create a vivid snapshot of one instance. This can be a happy and unexpected event, but it can also be something shocking.

Do you remember where you where when you first heard of Princess Diana's death? What were you doing when the news of the 9/11 bombings broke? Most people remember these memories in vivid detail, even though they were just doing something ordinary. Why is that? *Flashbulb* memories are memories that contain strong emotion. As a result, mundane events suddenly become more meaningful and you remember trivial details. But just because you remember the events doesn't mean that all the details you remember are correct. One man described how he was woken up early by an earthquake. However, reports show that the earthquake took place in the afternoon only!

Here are some tips on how you can focus on your happy memories:

✔ **Think happy.** Positive thinking – or thinking positive thoughts – can drive change in your life. With childhood memories the temptation as you grow older is to view events in a less than positive light. This may be the result of later life experiences, such as stressful events.

But don't let yourself do this. Instead of feeling sorry for yourself, think of ways in which an event made you a stronger and better person. You can also think of reasons why people did what they did. For example, a friend told me of how she was bullied at school, but as she got older, she realised what a difficult life the bully had and she stopped feeling sorry for herself and started counting her own blessings.

✔ **Scrapbooking is no scrappy task.** Forgetting what a great holiday you had is easy, especially as time moves on and you get more entrenched in the daily grind. But stopping and remembering what a wonderful time you had is important. Scrapbooking is a fun and great way to preserve precious memories. Many different websites give you guidelines and templates to get you started. Some people save tickets stubs to events they went to, brochures or postcards of places they visited, or even a leaf or flower from a park or hike that they loved. You can add all these mementos to your scrapbook. You can even buy special books and materials if you're feeling a little more creative in your efforts.

Many scrapbooking groups exist, so why not join one? You'll find that sharing your happy memories strengthens them in your mind, and you're more likely to remember them. In Chapter 11, I discuss the added benefits of socialising to keep your brain healthy.

✔ **Have a snack.** Think back on those lazy, sunny days when you didn't go to school and could spend all day at the park. Food can serve as a fantastic trigger for happy childhood memories because the taste and smell can remind you of a specific event. If you're missing your family and childhood friends, even thinking about the food you used to enjoy can boost your mood.

In Chapter 12, I list brain foods for a healthy life whatever your age.

If you were to sit down and list your top 20 memories, you may find that most of them are from your 20s and your 30s. This isn't unusual. Most people try things for the first time during this period and so tend to remember them more clearly. This may include first loves, books that sparked late-night debates, and first mortgages. This period is known as the *reminiscence bump* because a 'bump' or peak in the amount of memories that you can easily recall from this time exists.

# Using Your Everyday Knowledge: Semantic Memory

*Semantic memory* refers to your library of knowledge: bits of information that you've collected over the years – useless facts about the animal kingdom, treasured details about football statistics, even capital cities of countries you've visited. Think of semantic memory as your personal encyclopaedia or Wikipedia in your head.

 Look at this list of words and say out loud the first thing that comes to your mind.

> Bread – ?
>
> Dog – ?
>
> Tea – ?

You may have said the following pairs:

> Bread – butter
>
> Dog – cat
>
> Tea – coffee

What words you came up with isn't really significant because most people have a huge knowledge store to match the words in this example. If I asked you to tell me three things about a bird, you'd use information from your semantic memory to answer this question.

## Knowing the Eiffel Tower from the Leaning Tower

Learning facts about the world is something you never stop doing. Just because you're no longer at school, it doesn't mean you stop finding out about knowledge and information.

# Tell me a story

I sometimes work together with Dominic O'Brien, the eight-time winner of the World Memory Championships, who holds many titles in the *Guinness Book of World Records*. One amazing feat he performs is memorising 54 decks of playing cards in just a few hours!

Dominic uses a great illustration to create a bridge between new information and long-term knowledge (semantic memory). He usually uses a list of 10 to 15 words, but I'll just use 5 to describe the process – *bomb, helium, light, beryl, coal*. Most people struggle to remember all the words, and if they read them in the morning, by lunchtime only a handful can still recite even three words from the list.

Dominic tells the following story:

> You're asleep in your bed one night when you hear a loud explosion. It sounds like a **bomb**! Before you can do anything, you spot a **helium** balloon in the sky shining a bright **light** on the ground. You think that they're looking for the perpetrator. The light seems to be moving towards your room but instead it stops and shines on your neighbour **Beryl's** house. You start to worry that more bombs are going to start going off so you make your way out of the house and into the garden. Someone has left a large bag of **coal** in the middle of the walkway and you trip over it in the dark.

The story goes on and you can imagine that most people are drawn into it. To their amazement, they find that by the end of the day, they're able to remember the 15 words in the correct order and can even recite them backwards! The words in the list provide a clue to the first few elements in the periodic table: bomb (hydrogen), helium (helium), light (lithium), beryl (beryllium) and coal (carbon). Now you too can easily remember these words simply by thinking about the story.

Learning something new is a three-stage process:

- *Encoding* refers to how you represent the information in your memory.
- *Storage* is how you keep the information in your head.
- *Retrieval* is how you access the information when you need it.

Here are some tips to help you encode information better:

- **Picture this.** If you have to remember a list of new words, create a visual image in your mind instead of just repeating the words in your head. If you're at a party, don't just say someone's name to remind yourself. Think of what the person's wearing and think of where she was standing when you met her. All these visual cues help trigger your memory when you have to remember the person's name at a later date. In Chapter 7, I list more strategies to help you remember names and faces.

✔ **Make it deep.** It's easier just to remember something new by looking at something superficial or shallow, such as what the word looks like or even what it sounds like. You may be tempted to remember as little as possible to get by. But this method won't help much at all. Instead, think of what something means, what rhymes with it – anything that makes you think about the information in a more meaningful way makes the information stick in your head.

✔ **Organise, organise, organise.** Has anyone ever told you, 'I already said it so many times, why can't you remember?' Everyone knows the feeling – you can hear something over and over again and yet never remember it! But you can change that. Create a framework to help you organise new information. When you read something, think of your framework and attach what you're reading to your framework. It helps you remember the contents of what you read much better.

✔ **Create a connection.** Link new information to something you already know. Don't just list the new information that you're learning, but think carefully about how you can connect it to something you know well. If you're learning a new history fact, think of an event with which you're familiar and create a link between the new and familiar historical facts. This process – called *semantic linking* – can help you retrieve the information later on.

Just repeating something is unlikely to help you remember. You need to make the information meaningful if you want to remember it. If you think of student days, this may explain why late-night cramming before exams doesn't help very much! When you elaborate on what you're learning using the strategies listed in the preceding bulleted list, you'll be more successful at encoding the information for recall later.

In the section 'Making associations that last', later in this chapter, I list ways for better storage.

## Making associations that last

Why do you forget things? The first comfort you can find is that forgetting is simply the natural course of information – items in your memory decay over time, just like food left outside. Another reason you forget is that when you learn something new, you can confuse it with something old. If the information is similar, then it's easier to get confused. A third possibility for why you forget is because you can't remember 'where' you stored the information.

## Where you are matters

A diving instructor was puzzled because his divers kept forgetting objects that they'd found underwater, even when he asked the divers about the objects shortly after they were back on dry land. To find out why this was the case, some psychologists conducted an experiment with divers.

The psychologists gave one group of underwater divers a list of words to learn underwater and gave another group a list to learn on land. They then tested the divers' memories of the word list both on land and underwater.

The group that learned the list underwater remembered the list much better in the water but struggled to remember it on land. In contrast, the group who learned the list on land had better memories on land but forgot the list when they were underwater.

This story is a great example of how remembering where you were when you learned the information can boost your memory.

Use the following tips to help you remember where you left that information that keeps escaping your memory:

- ✔ **Contextualise.** The context in which you hear information is a powerful trigger to unlock your memory. If you're struggling to remember something, go back to the place where you first heard or read the information. At work, go back to the room where you stood and recreate the scenario to trigger your memory. If a friend gave you some important information to remember, go back to the café or restaurant where you had that conversation. (For a detailed example, see the nearby sidebar 'Where you are matters'.)

- ✔ **Remember your state.** The mood that you were in when you learned the information also acts as a trigger to help you remember. If you were in a good mood when you first heard about a new project in which you were involved, try to think about those same emotions. In Chapter 9, I look at ways in which a positive mindset can keep your brain healthy.

- ✔ **Take a trip.** The *journey method* – a way to link new information to a mental picture of something familiar – is a trick some memory experts use. Here's an example: imagine you've just woken up and you see a poster of John Travolta on your cupboard. You remember that your friend gave it to you because you liked the movie *Grease*. You go into the bathroom and notice your unfinished school project – a model of the Eiffel Tower – is lying unfinished in the middle of the floor. You drowsily make your way to the living room and see that your brother has spilled pasta sauce all over the couch.

The story goes on to help you remember the countries in the European Union. I have only listed three of the countries (Greece, France, and Italy), but by using the journey method, you can remember all 27 of them!

*Proactive interference* is when old information that you know makes it harder to remember new information. An example of proactive interference is when you get a new PIN number for your credit card, but you keep using your old number instead. *Retroactive interference* is when something new makes you forget something you were previously thinking about. An example is when you forget where you're going because you stop to look for your car keys.

Still struggling? Use cues to trigger your memory. Imagine that you're learning new vocabulary words in Spanish (I list the words in English): *shoes, hat, belt, shirt, trousers, chair, table, desk, lamp*. First, group the items that belong together and then think of category headings to help you retrieve this information. Studies have found that when you use category cues, like *clothes* and *furniture*, for this example, you're twice as likely to remember all the words associated with the category. You can try this with any group of items like colours or eating utensils (like *fork, spoon,* and *knife*).

Did you ever get the feeling that you know what something is but you just can't get the right words to say it? I discuss how to avoid the *tip-of-the-tongue phenomenon* in Chapter 6.

---

# 50 First Dates

You may remember a quirky movie called *50 First Dates* about a woman, played by Drew Barrymore, who's lost her ability to form long-term memories. Although this storyline may seem far-fetched, it's sadly the case that some people do suffer memory loss like this as the result of a brain injury. Consider the story of 47-year-old Michelle. As a result of two car accidents, all her memories before 1994 have been 'erased' and she has no recollection of them. Her long-suffering husband has to show her their wedding photos daily to remind her of what they share.

To complicate things for Michelle, she's unable to convert daily experiences in her short-term memory (see Chapter 5) to long-term memory. This means that it's not unusual for her to leave the house only to forget where she's going. She relies on technology like satellite-navigation systems to get her to places just half a mile from her house. Michelle describes each day as a new day with no memory of what she experienced the day before. Although she loves certain TV programmes, she can't remember all the characters and can't follow any of the plot lines. She's upbeat, though, and says that at least she feels that she's never seen the same show twice.

# Long-term Skills: Procedural Memory

Can you describe how you tie your shoelace? You may struggle, though you'd probably have no difficulty if you actually had a shoe in your hand and had to get ready to go out. Why is it so difficult to give a step-by-step breakdown for simple tasks that some people do every day, like tying a shoelace, driving a car, or even writing your name? My 3-year-old son, on the other hand, has no difficulty in telling me how to do a simple task step-by-step. He's learning how to write his name, and he spends a lot of time on each step. For example, when he's writing the letter *M*, he says out loud, 'Up the hill, down the hill, up the hill and down the hill.' I'm sure that you wouldn't spend as much time writing the letter *M*!

*Procedural memory* refers to the skills that you have that are automatic – things that you no longer have to spend much time thinking about, like writing letters or tying a tie. Your brain remembers what to do without actually keeping track of each step. That's why it's often hard to list each step. The question is, how do you learn a new thing so it becomes procedural memory and you no longer have to think so hard about it? For example, you may be trying to learn a new language or perfect a dish.

The following sections offer tips to transfer that new information into a long-lasting memory.

## Practising for perfection

I heard someone say, 'Practice only makes perfect if practice is perfect.' That statement holds much truth. When you do something over and over again, you're training both your brain and your muscles to remember it. Athletes refer to this as *muscle memory (see Chapter 7)*, where you do an action automatically because your muscles 'remember', like riding a bicycle or skating. The practice statement is important because if you don't learn something correctly the first time, your body has to unlearn the incorrect way first before it can learn a new and better way of doing something.

Think of how you hold a pencil. I remember my teacher being very strict with all her students, and we could only hold the pencil one way or we'd get in trouble. That pencil-holding technique has stuck with me, and I find it very uncomfortable to hold a pencil any other way. This is true for a lot of other activities. For example, if you like skiing and decide to take some lessons despite having skied already for a number of years, you may be surprised to discover that your posture and form aren't good. Your instructor has to work harder to get you to change your form than if she was teaching a novice skier. This is because your muscles have stored a certain way of skiing that you now have to unlearn in order to learn the correct form. So the next time you're learning something new, make sure that it's the correct way the first time around. This way you won't have to learn it twice!

The power of rewards in improving memory is known as the *law of effect*. This law is very simple – if you receive something enjoyable as a result of learning something new, you're more likely to repeat the behaviour that caused you to learn. As a child, these rewards may be gold stickers or a good grade on an exam. As an adult, this may be praise from a loved one or even a promotion at work. But another side to the law of effect exists – if you receive something negative, such as criticism or disappointment, as a result of learning something new, you're less likely to repeat that behaviour.

Reward yourself! Gold stars and colourful stickers aren't just for the classroom. Set up a reward system when you're trying to learn something new. Break down the information into smaller chunks and each time you're successful at learning a chunk give yourself a 'sticker'. After you've successfully completed the task, treat yourself to the reward you set – a new dress, a short holiday. The treat doesn't have to cost money; it can also be a special day with friends. The goal is to create incentives to train your brain to absorb the information and associate positive emotions with the learning process. This method not only makes learning more pleasurable, but it also helps you remember the information for much longer. As a bonus, when you think back on your reward or look at photos of the event, this serves as a trigger to help you remember the information that you learned.

Many famous athletes have a little routine that they do before a game. Maybe they tie their laces a certain way or sleep in their uniform the night before a big game. One major league hockey player stuck his hockey stick in the toilet before each game! Such superstitions aren't uncommon among athletes. Although these routines do very little to help create connections in memory that last, some people think that repeating familiar routines can help to reduce anxiety before an important performance or activity.

You may have your own superstitions about doing something before a date or a presentation or even an important meeting. But it's far more productive to think of positive actions that are directly related to the event, rather than something unrelated. For example, before a date, think of questions that you want to ask the person (not in an interrogative way!); before a presentation, think of the key points that you want to get across; and before an important meeting, think of three things you want to communicate about yourself or your work and how you're going to do that.

## Training in your sleep

Sleep is a great booster when you learn. Having a rest after learning something strengthens the information that you learned. Think of your school days. Remember those multiple choice exams? They look so easy yet they can be so confusing if more than one choice seems like the right answer! Many situations in daily life can confuse people. For example, you may forget whether you turned off the oven when you're on your way out the door.

Not only does sleep improve memory, but you also make fewer errors in working on a task. When you sleep, your brain uses this time to recharge and separate real events and factual information from information that's not correct. As a result, not only are you more refreshed, but you're less likely to get confused and forget whether you left the oven on. In Chapter 14, I talk more about the power of sleep in recharging your brain and making learning stick.

When musicians try to memorise a piece of music, they don't just play a song over and over again. They get their brain involved too. You may be wondering why. The reason is simple. If all musicians do is play a song over and over again, their muscles learn the movement, but if they get distracted partway through the song, it's harder for them to pick up and carry on playing. In fact, some people have to start all over from the beginning because they can't just pick up playing from a random point in the song.

You don't have to be an amazing musician to benefit from musicians' techniques. When you're learning something new or have to do something you're nervous about, such as giving a presentation at work, get your brain involved too by focusing carefully on what you need to do. First, get rid of distractions. Next, instead of just giving your presentation over and over again out loud, you can also give it in your head. Go over different questions that your colleagues may ask you. Finally, stop and think about your answers to these questions when you're halfway through the presentation. And then pick up from where you stopped and continue your presentation.

# Chapter 5

# Improving Your Short-Term Memory

*In This Chapter*

▶ Boosting your verbal memory

▶ Keeping your visual memory intact with easy tricks

▶ Using your spatial memory more

*Y*ou're meeting some friends after work and one of them introduces you to a new person. After exchanging names and spending the evening sharing similar interests, you make plans to keep in touch. The man gives you his phone number, but you realise that you don't have a paper or pencil, or even your Blackberry with you. 'Never mind,' you say. 'I can remember it.' After repeating the phone number a few times to yourself, you head home. Sensibly, you decide to jot down the number as soon as you head in the door. Too late! You can't remember the last four digits.

Short-term memory is the space that you have to hold information for a short time. You can think of short-term memory like a holding zone – you won't keep the information in your short-term memory for long, just long enough until you can transfer the information to a piece of paper, your computer, or even your long-term memory store.

This chapter looks at how you can train three types of short-term memory – verbal, visual, and spatial. Although you may sometimes use these types of memory together, you usually tend to focus on one at a time.

# Speaking Your Brain's Language: Verbal Memory

*Verbal short-term memory* refers to language and information that you hear.

Ask someone to read out the following letters while you try to remember them.

NBCUSAATM

How did you do? Were you able to remember all nine letters in the correct order? You may have figured out that you can break up these letters to look like this:

NBC – USA – ATM

You can see that each unit represents a very common acronym. This probably made it a lot easier for you to remember the letters.

Now try this one. I've broken it into smaller sections for you.

CRM – BRD – UAL

You may have found this example more difficult. Even breaking the letters down into smaller sections may not have helped. You may be wondering why. The small sections may not have helped because the acronyms were unfamiliar. This is what they mean:

CRM: Customer Relationship Management

BRD: Biological Resource Division

UAL: United Airlines

Did knowing what the acronyms mean help you remember the letters? It may not have, because here again the meanings may have been unfamiliar.

If you find it difficult to remember phone numbers and more than ten new names, you can comfort yourself with the knowledge that, on average, most people can only remember seven pieces of information at a single time. A *piece* of information can refer to one number or one word, or even one instruction. When you group information together, such as in the example with the letters (NBC – USA – ATM), each group counts as one piece of information so you only have to remember three pieces of information. This process of 'chunking' or grouping information together is the reason why you may be able to recall a shorter landline local number, but not a longer mobile number.

A common expression when discussing the limits of short-term memory is 'seven plus or minus two'. This means that a few people can remember up to nine pieces of information, but most remember seven. You can think of this expression as a golden rule for verbal short-term memory.

So how can you boost your verbal short-term memory? In this section, I give you strategies and tips to do just that.

## *Articulating for a better brain*

You can boost your verbal short-term memory skills in many ways. Here are some tried-and-tested tips:

- ✔ **Time matters.** *When* you hear information affects how well you remember it. For example, you remember information at the beginning of a list better than words presented in the middle of a list because you're able to rehearse them more. This is known as the *primacy effect*. Also, you best remember items at the end of a list, even more than those words at the beginning of the list, because you've just heard them and so don't need to remember them for very long. This is known as the *recency effect*. So if someone gives you a long list of things to do, break it down into many lists to avoid the 'slump' in the middle of the list.

- ✔ **Turn down the distractions.** An unrelated thought springing to mind, an interruption by someone else, or another distraction within the environment, such as a telephone ringing or a child crying, is often sufficient to erase the contents of verbal short-term memory. This is because unless you continue to pay attention to the contents of short-term memory, they decay very rapidly and are soon lost for good. Placing yourself in situations that minimise likely distractions is very important if you're going to make effective use of working memory. Background noise also plays a role in how much material you can remember. Silence is much more conducive to good verbal short-term memory. If you're trying to remember some important information, you may find that turning down the music helps!

- ✔ **Focus on one thing.** Activities that require you to switch your attention from one thing to another can speed up how fast you forget something. The act of switching or *multitasking* can overload you and result in you forgetting even simple things.

You may find yourself standing at top of your stairs thinking, 'What was I up here for?' Doing too many things at the same time means that you can't do one thing well. So cut back – do one task at a time and you'll find yourself better at remembering things at work and at home.

✔ **Know your limits.** Avoid overloading your memory by giving yourself bite-sized chunks of information to remember. Remembering the information that you were asked to remember is more important than trying to prove yourself as the next memory champion by keeping a long string of information in your head.

## Talking fast to remember more

You may think of a fast talker as a smooth operator or someone who's trying to scam you by selling you something you really don't need. Actually, talking fast can do wonders for your verbal short-term memory.

Saying information that you need to remember over and over again can help you remember what you need. But keep in mind two things:

✔ **Length counts.** The length of a word makes a big difference in how well you can remember it. Look at these words: *refrigerator, hippopotamus, Mississippi, aluminium*. You're more likely to forget them compared to words that you can repeat more easily, such as *bus, clock, spoon,* and *fish*. The longer it takes to repeat or rehearse something, the harder it is to remember. This is known as the *word length effect,* which means that longer words are harder to remember. To boost your memory of longer words, ask to look at a list, rather than just listen to it.

✔ **Sounds matter.** A list of words that are distinct (such as *bus, clock, spoon, fish, mouse*) are much easier to remember than a list of words that sound very similar (rhyming words such as *man, cat, map, mat, can, cap*). When things sound similar, you're more likely to get confused and forget what you need to do. So if you're trying to remember your shopping list, group your items by categories (dairy, meat, breads), rather than alphabetically.

Here's a sure-fire way to boost your verbal memory. Listen to two different sounds: a high pitch and a low pitch. Then decide whether they're the same. Try it with different sounds. Musicians train this skill. Teachers also use this technique to boost skills in people who find it hard to discriminate different sounds when they're learning a new language. (See Chapter 15 for more games to boost your verbal memory.)

## Speed it up!

Psychologists found that talking fast can make a difference in retaining information. Look at these lists of words:

Four – six – four – seven

Pedwar – chwech – pedwar – saith

The first list takes a lot less time to say than the second list. Does this affect verbal short-term memory?

Psychologists found that the English-speaking children who were given the first list of numbers had much higher scores in remembering the list than the second group. They gave the second list of numbers (in Welsh) to students in Wales. Their scores were much lower.

This was very puzzling until the psychologists realised that speed does matter! It took the Welsh students much longer to say the numbers in Welsh, which affected their scores. After they took the speed of saying the numbers out of the equation, no difference between the two groups of children existed.

# Seeing Your Brain's Perspective: Visual Memory

*Visual short-term memory* deals with images, such as photos and pictures – information that's hard to say. You use visual short-term memory to recognise places you've been, photos you've seen, and images you need to store mentally.

Try your visual short-term memory on the test shown in Figure 5-1. Look at the image and then cover up the image and look at the empty grid in Figure 5-2.

On Figure 5-2, point to where the dots were on the grid in the correct order that they were shown in Figure 5-1. How many dots can you remember? Most adults can remember about three or four dots in the correct order.

Visual short-term memory doesn't last very long. Yet it's quite resistant to distraction. When you were looking at Figure 5-2, you probably blinked several times, looked away to check something else out, and maybe even let your mind drift to another thought. But you did quite well at remembering the locations on the grid in Figure 5-2 because your eyes take a 'snapshot' of what they see, and your brain stores that image. Your brain doesn't save the image for long though, or transfer it to long-term memory, which explains why you find it easier to recognise someone new that same day than a few days later.

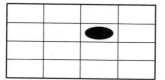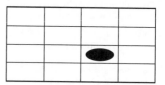

**Figure 5-1:** An example of a visual short-term memory test – part one.

**Figure 5-2:** An example of a visual short-term memory test – part two.

 Visual short-term memory skills are usually slightly weaker than verbal short-term memory ones. This means that you find it easier to remember words, numbers, and verbal information than to remember images. One explanation for this is that you use language much more than you use your memory for images.

In Chapter 7, I discuss how visual memory is excellent when you're young, but as you start to learn language your brain uses this skill less and so you lose some of this ability. Chapter 7 provides ways in which you can keep your visual memory sharp whatever your age.

# Harnessing the power of visualisation

*Visualisation* is a powerful tool, and you can easily underestimate its effectiveness. Numerous studies show that the brain responds to visualisation in the same way as it does to physical practice.

Psychologists divided basketball players into three groups. They asked one group to practise shooting baskets daily; another group to only visualise shooting baskets, but not actually practise; and a final group to do nothing at all. After a month the psychologists tested the basketball skills of all three groups. As you may guess, the people who'd done nothing did really poorly and seemed to have lost some of their skills. The people who'd been practising diligently for the last month improved their skills by 24 per cent. But what's most surprising is that the people who'd just visualised shooting baskets also improved their skills to almost the same level as those who were actually practising!

Not convinced yet? A Harvard study found that people who visualised playing the piano activated the same part of the brain as those who actually practised the piano.

Here are some pointers for how to harness the power of visualisation in your own life:

- ✔ **Close your eyes.** Sometimes this can help you block out distractions around you and focus just on what you want to remember. Is it someone's face? A map? Close your eyes and imagine the image in your head.

- ✔ **Draw it out.** If you're a list-writer, here's a twist you can do. Instead of writing down what you need to do – for example, if you've invited friends over for a Sunday roast and you need to remind yourself of what to do, such as thaw the meat or buy potatoes and carrots – why not draw it? It'll probably be a lot quicker and the picture may even make you smile when you see it. Another way to visualise things is to make a graph or a diagram. You may prefer to represent everything you need to do to prepare for your Sunday dinner as a diagram. First take out meat and then season it, and so on.

- ✔ **Write it out.** Keep in mind that visualising doesn't just mean pictures or images. If you're the type of person who needs to see things written out, don't change that. Keep writing down what you need to remember. Just keep the information accessible and visible so you don't waste mental energy trying to remember where you left your list!

Some people find it useful to leave their list near their task, so you could place a shopping list on the fridge door, directions to a party near your car keys, and a list of errands for the day in your coat pocket. Put your list in a meaningful location right away. Chances are, if you wait until later, you'll forget where you left your list.

✔ **Be an imaginary teacher.** If you're trying to remember some particularly difficult information, perhaps when revising for a course or a presentation at work, imagine yourself teaching the information to an imaginary audience. Visualising yourself giving your presentation ahead of time can have the same impact as practising it over and over again. This technique is particularly useful if you don't have a lot of time to yourself or if you travel to and from work. Use this time to visualise yourself in front of your colleagues, going over each aspect of your presentation. Try to visualise yourself answering questions as well and you'll find that this helps you make the process of giving the presentation and anticipating questions more automatic.

When you're trying to remember faces, create a visual association. Think of an association to help a new colleague's name, perhaps a prominent feature like big eyes or a small nose. Now picture it on a location, maybe Jim's nose on a canapé plate if you were eating a canapé when you were introduced to him. By creating a connection between a visual feature (the nose on a canapé plate) and verbal information (Jim's name), you're increasing your chances of remembering that information.

## Photographing your memory

You may have heard of people who have a photographic memory – they look at something once and they can remember it. This skill is something that less than 10 per cent of people have. It's most evident in childhood, but as language skills develop people lose their ability to create 'snapshots' of what they see.

*Iconic memory* is the term that describes a very quick visual image. Your eyes store images in less than a second, and if I showed you a picture for half a second, the image would remain in 'your mind's eye', although you may not even be aware of it. The iconic memory doesn't last very long, though, and you can quickly forget it.

Here's a quick way to train your photographic memory. If you enjoy reading different online blogs, you may have noticed that some of them have *tag clouds* – visual descriptions of different topics included on that blog. Figure 5-3 shows you an example of a tag cloud. Some words are in larger text than others to illustrate which topics the blogger discusses more often. If you read that blog regularly, train yourself to recognise changes in the size of the text in the tag clouds. Look at the text for a couple of seconds only, then close your eyes and try to decide which text has 'grown' since you last read the blog. (See Chapter 7 for more games to boost your visual memory.)

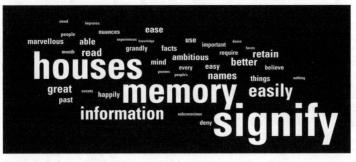

**Figure 5-3:** An example of a tag cloud.

 If you have to remember to do something, bring up a photograph in your mind. For example, you need to bring a cake to the Christmas party. Think of a photo with a cake in it from last year's party. It's much more memorable than repeating your list of errands over and over to yourself.

# Moving at Your Brain's Pace: Spatial Memory

*Spatial short-term memory* relates to how well you can recall locations and directions.

 Use your right hand and tap out a square on the table in front of you. Do this a few times. Now do it without looking at your hand and go as fast as you can without making any mistakes. So far so good? Now take your left hand and draw circles in the air. How is your right hand doing? Any mistakes? You may have already given up by now. You may be wondering why you found this simple activity quite difficult.

You use the same part of your brain to plan and control your movements. When you attempt two different activities at the same time, it gets difficult because you have to process two different movements simultaneously. Individuals with motor difficulties find it especially hard to do this type of activity.

You use different parts of your brain to remember verbal and spatial information. So if you're trying to remember directions, why not draw it out instead of writing it? This way if you're distracted by someone talking, you're less likely to forget what you're doing. In Chapter 7, I provide strategies to help you remember directions.

## Getting a bird's eye perspective

Spatial memory works best when you can look from above, like a bird, rather than looking around you. Check out these tips on how to achieve a bird's eye perspective to keep your spatial memory sharp:

✔ **Change shoes.** I recently gave a friend who was new in town directions to a café. When she still hadn't shown up an hour later I started to worry. Imagine my surprise when I found out that she'd walked in the opposite direction from my instructions, despite my giving her many landmarks. It was only then that I realised how different spatial perspectives can get you lost. People often give directions from their viewpoint.

This can result in a lot of frustration when you try to follow what the person is saying. Next time, put yourself in the other person's shoes – see it from her perspective.

✔ **Walk the walk.** The next time someone gives you directions, adopt an ego-moving perspective while he's talking. Imagine yourself walking through that route in your head. Make that right turn, stop at the traffic light, turn down that second street and mentally scan for his house. When you actually make that journey, you've already done it once in your head. Now you have no excuse for getting lost! Chapter 7 has more tips for remembering directions.

✔ **Look down.** It helps to view locations and directions in a grid-like way. Try to create an aerial view of where you are and where you need to go. People who do this have a much better sense of direction. Imagine that you're a bird and flying over the next few streets that you walk down. How would the streets look? Where would you turn? This strategy of creating an aerial perspective can also help you find your way back from your destination to your original starting point. Even if you haven't been to the area you're in before, creating an aerial view from what you do know about the area (such as a street or a landmark) helps you to navigate better.

## See my world

Researchers often use computer games to understand how spatial memory works. One great way to examine this is to ask people to experience different types of virtual environments. Some people see objects moving towards them and others see them moving through the virtual environment. The first perspective is known as an *object-moving perspective* where you're stationary and watch objects come toward you – for example, while waiting at a bus stop. Think of a third-person adventure game, where you move relative to the objects around you. The second perspective is known as the *ego-moving perspective* where you're moving and passing by objects – for example, walking down a street past shops, houses, and parked cars or in a room past tables and chairs. Think of a first-person, car-racing game, where objects around you are moving relative to your position.

This difference in perspective impacts how well you understand spatial language, like directions. For example, if a friend tells you to pick up the 'front book' from a row of books, does he mean the book in front of you or in front of him? That depends on your perspective. In the object-moving perspective, you'd probably pick up the book closest to you. However, in the ego-moving perspective, you'd pick up the book farthest away from you.

Language is flexible and doesn't always make sense. Many words are ambiguous, just like the example of *front* that I use in this sidebar. Your spatial perspective can make a big difference in how you understand what someone's saying. Field studies show that spatial perspective changes during travel. People who are about to begin a journey are more likely to have an ego-moving perspective. The same is true for those who've just completed a trip. Those people in the middle of their journey view the world from an object-moving perspective.

Video games tend to polarise thinking: some argue that they're a waste of time, but others insist that they're a worthy relaxation tool. Now the pro-video gamers can take comfort in the knowledge that gamers tend to have better visual-spatial skills than non-gamers. They're much faster not only in the game they love playing, but also in other unrelated tasks that measure how quickly you can solve a problem. Sceptics used to think that a trade-off existed: to gain speed, you lose accuracy. However, research now shows that this isn't the case. Gamers are faster and also remain accurate because they develop their skills to use their visual-spatial skills better through video games. So if you want to improve your visual-spatial skills, maybe it's time to hit the video game shop!

## *Move through space*

If you've ever had the pleasure of talking to an animated and excited young child, you probably noticed how often he moved about while he spoke. One thing that children frequently do is mirror the actions of one hand with the other. Ask a child to count using his fingers. A young child often raises his fingers on both hands. You can see this action, known as *mirror movements,* not just with hands, but also with toes and feet. In this section, I discuss how different movements can help your spatial memory. Chapter 14 lists ways to get moving to keep your brain and body fit.

It's very uncommon for adults to show *mirror movements.* Those who do this find that they can't move one side of the body without moving the other. Scientists have now discovered that a cross-over exists. When the brain sends a message to the limbs to move, it sends it to both sides, instead of just one. Although very few people suffer from this difficulty, the knowledge gives an important clue for how the brain works to move the body.

Here are some tips on how to use actions to help your memory:

✔ **Mirror, mirror.** Look at Figure 5-4. Can you guess whether the object on the right is a mirror image of the one on the left? Your skills at mentally rotating an object are linked to spatial memory.

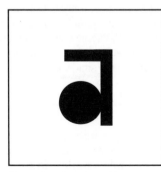 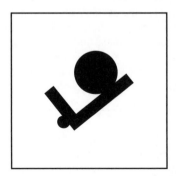

**Figure 5-4:** Rotating objects.

✔ **Move your marbles!** I used to love playing with marbles when I was younger. My favourite thing about them was the way the colours in the glass shimmered in the sunlight. Even today when I see marbles I think back on happy, carefree days as a child. Marbles can also make you feel good as an adult. Psychologists found that a simple thing like moving marbles up into a higher box is more likely to make you think of positive memories. However, when you move marbles down into a lower box, you remember more negative or sad experiences. Why is this? The language people use to describe emotions is closely linked with spatial movements: 'I'm on top of the world', or 'I feel down today'. When you move marbles up, that action triggers words that describe forward motion, which in turn triggers good feelings. So the next time you're feeling down, start moving marbles up.

To boost your spatial memory, don't just think of the route to get to a place. Find out what landmarks are present along your journey and create a mental map of the path you take with those landmarks present as well. The combination of a mental map of the route matched with visual landmarks boosts your spatial memory.

# Chapter 6

# Improving Your Language Skills

In This Chapter
▶ Boosting your verbal skills
▶ Using easy tricks to keep your language intact

L anguage is one of the first skills you learn. From infancy, coos and aahs are early steps in communicating with those around you. These cute early sounds are known as babbling because they represent babies trying out new sounds that they've heard. Babies develop these skills and begin using one word coupled with actions to let others know their intentions. For example, an 18-month-old will point to a bottle of milk and say 'Mi-mi' to express her desires. Language develops at an impressive rate, with children learning hundreds of new words in the first few years of their lives.

As you get older, language skills get more sophisticated. You can speak freely to express your ideas, debate with friends on topics of interest, and share your feelings with loved ones. What a shock when you slowly discover that this wonderful gift of language starts breaking down in adulthood. But it doesn't have to be this way. In this chapter, you discover how you can keep your language skills intact.

## Avoiding Verbal Loss

Searching for the right word in the middle of a conversation can be frustrating. However, you don't need to find yourself in a situation where you're searching for the right word. You can do several things to avoid this problem.

# Banishing the tip-of-the-tongue phenomenon

Everyone struggles with the *tip-of-the-tongue phenomenon* (TOT for short) – when you can describe a word in detail but you just can't remember what it is.

Here's how TOT works. I'm thinking of a fruit, I ate it for breakfast, it's juicy and I can see it in my head but I just can't remember what it's called. Two hours later, the name pops in my head while I'm in the middle of a meeting – I was thinking of a pomegranate. This example is simple – you're more commonly searching for words you say less frequently, but you can see that it's not always easy for someone to guess what you're thinking of from your description.

Communicating something that you can see in your mind and almost taste so vividly, yet can't remember the name of, is frustrating. Sometimes it's even harder to describe what you want because another word is 'stuck' in your mind. In my example, all I could think about was a pear instead of an orange! You're searching for the word but just can't find it. Why did I keep thinking of a pear and was it stopping me from thinking about an orange? Actually, thinking about a pear was my brain's way of helping me think of orange. My brain tried to find related words, such as the names of other juicy fruits, to trigger the missing word.

Psychologists describe this as a temporary breakdown in your mental dictionary: you can think of the meaning of the word but not what it sounds like. You store information in different parts of your brain. You store images – for example, the picture of an orange – in one part of the brain, and the related meaning, such as a description of an orange, recipes using oranges and the taste of an orange, in another part of the brain. With TOT, it's as if the bridge connecting your images and your words is broken.

It may be that you haven't been using this connection very often and so it becomes weak. Some say it's like an overgrown bike path – once it was smooth and clear, but because you haven't used it very often weeds and grass grow over the path and it becomes harder to see where the path is. As you get older, these connections also get weaker. Everyone experiences TOT, but often it happens with words that you don't use very often.

People's names are also hard to remember because it is arbitrary. The name 'Tracy' doesn't not necessarily remind you of something specific and so it is easy to forget the association between a name and a face if we don't attach something meaningful to the name, such as 'my childhood friend'.

Everyone experiences TOT. Although it may be annoying or even frustrating, it's not something you should panic about. One reason people struggle with TOT is that as they get older people seldom use the 'path' that connects different information such as images and descriptions.

## Using a variety of words

Don't get stuck in a rut, using the same words and same ideas every day. In order to avoid TOT, keeping the connections active is important. The more often you use language and seek out opportunities to use language creatively, the less likely you are to experience TOT.

Here are some suggestions that can help:

✔ **Play games with yourself.** Set yourself a target – for example, name as many animals as you can in 30 seconds. Try to name one animal per second. Now make it harder – name as many animals as you can that start with the letter *B* in 30 seconds. Try a different topic, maybe fruit or furniture. You can add more time on if you find it too easy, or pick harder letters. The goal of this game is to challenge your mind to create connections between items in a category. Also try to think of words you may not use very often. You may even find yourself making a mental store of animal names when you read the newspaper!

✔ **Do crosswords.** Crosswords are a fun and fantastic way to keep those connections alive! If you're not a big fan of crosswords, start with something easy and on a topic that you enjoy, perhaps gardening or travel. Crosswords are very effective in combating TOT because they give you a clue and you have to search for the word in your mind (see Chapter 15 for crossword puzzles that you can do).

✔ **Give yourself clues.** If you're a list-writer, here's a technique you can try. Instead of writing down what you need to do – for example, take out the chicken from the freezer, get rosemary from the garden, buy carrots – why not write out in clues? So here's what my list may look like: take out the 'bird' from the freezer; in the garden get the herb that starts with the name of a flower; buy a vegetable that's supposed to give you great eyesight. By doing this, you're giving yourself descriptions that force you to think of the word. But you may not want to do this if you're giving the list to someone else!

✔ **Keep a diary.** This is a proven way to keep your language skills intact. You can just write a little every day, but try to use words that you wouldn't usually use and be as descriptive as possible.

Imagine yourself as the next Dan Brown and try to write about your day as if it's a detective story or even a romance if you prefer. The goal is challenge your mind to think about your day and to use language in a creative way.

✔ **Finish your thoughts.** And finally, always finish your thoughts. Sometimes it's easier to let someone guess what you want to say so you start saying something but then trail off at the end. Try to avoid this. Even if it takes you a little longer, finishing your thoughts is an important habit to establish. You need to be active in communicating your ideas if you want to keep the 'path' between images and descriptions clear.

# Remembering Your Shopping List and Other Important Things

How many times have you found yourself standing in the middle of an aisle full of food scratching your head and trying to remember what you needed for dinner that night, or suddenly stopping while driving somewhere because you couldn't remember where you were going? This happens to everyone. People have busy lives and sometimes some things like shopping lists or where you're supposed to go gets pushed to the back of your priority list.

Don't worry too much about this! The problem arises when this happens all the time rather than just occasionally. If you're regularly forgetful in this way, this section includes some tips to help.

## Repeating, repeating, repeating

People sometimes forget that repetition can be a powerful tool to move something into their long-term memory (which is the permanent memory). But a knack to using repetition exists.

Here are a few guidelines:

✔ **Repeat only for a short time.** You don't need to spend hours repeating something like a topic you want to remember. In fact, if you spend too long doing this you'll overtire yourself and likely give up altogether! Instead, spend just a few minutes going over in your head what you want to remember.

✔ **Repeat what you want to remember periodically.** You don't have to do this at a set time every day – in fact, it's better if you do it at different times. For example, while you're brushing your teeth, go over what you want to remember in your head. The next day, do this while you're getting dressed. When you repeat information at varying times, you tell your brain that this information is important, and it creates a strong connection that you'll remember for a long time.

✔ **When you repeat information, don't forget to say the list from the beginning.** Often you may only repeat things at the end of your list or even out of order. This isn't a good way to train your memory and you'll end up forgetting things more often than not. Train yourself to repeat things in the order you hear them and from the beginning of the list and you'll notice a big difference.

## *Rhyming to remember*

Your brain stores information using different clues. One clue uses *phonological information* – this simply means the way the word sounds. Your brain makes a connection between words that sound the same and these words are activated when you're trying to think of another word (see the earlier section 'Banishing the tip-of-the-tongue phenomenon' for more on this). This can explain why when you are trying to say 'pear', all you can think about is 'bear', or why you think someone's name is 'Diane' when it's actually 'Donna'. The fact that our brains makes a connection between words that sound the same makes rhyming words such a great trigger for remembering things.

Another clue that our brain uses is *semantic information* – information about the word, such as the category it belongs to and what it's used for. Think of your long-term memory as a big library. Your filing system for words has categories, such as fruit, furniture, and animals. You may have a more detailed filing system that also divides each category into small and more specific categories, such as pets, wild animals, animals that fly, and animals that swim. You can use this system to stop you forgetting important dates, appointments, and meetings.

Many great tips exist for remembering information when you don't have a paper and pencil in hand. One tip is to try to create an association and to link it with another word. Choosing rhyming words is a good technique because your brain remembers words that sound similar. If you put them to music, the words become even more memorable. For example, if you have a doctor's appointment, you can make up a rhyme like 'See Dr Brown in town'. The rhymes that you make up can even be silly or nonsensical; that helps the words to be more memorable (think of the *Jabberwocky*).

Another tip is to remember words in categories. If you're trying to remember your shopping list, think of all the items that you can find in the dairy aisle and then think of all the meat products, and so on. If you have a meeting and you need to remember several key points, organise them in categories. This helps you to remember more information than if you just kept a running tab of all your ideas for the meeting in your head.

Don't forget to repeat the information to yourself. Just coming up with a rhyme or an organiser style isn't enough to ensure that you remember. You need to repeat the information a few times to yourself to make sure that the connection is strong.

# Measuring Your Language Skills with Verbal IQ Tests

You may think that you're losing your language skills, but it's difficult to know how true this actually is without having the ability to measure your skills against someone else's. Psychologists use many different types of tests to measure how the brain works, including language skills.

The benefit of verbal IQ tests is that they're based on thousands of people from different backgrounds and experiences and provide an excellent representation for what language should be. For example, verbal IQ tests reveal what language ability should be in your 20s, 30s, 40s, 50s, 60s, 70s, 80s and so on. So you don't have to guess how good your skills are – you can measure them using an objective test.

## Looking at verbal IQ tests

The purpose of verbal IQ tests is to measure your language skills. If you haven't already guessed, your mastery of language is important in everything you do. You show the signs of getting older or even feeling stressed in your language. You start to forget simple words, and lose the thread of conversation and even family member's names.

So how do you know when this behaviour is the result of being over-tired or stressed out and not the start of a downhill pattern? That's when IQ tests come in. They measure how well you use language to express your thoughts and understand ideas and conversations with other people. Most IQ tests ask you to complete a range of different activities and you can see examples of these in the next section.

## IQ tests of the past

You may have come across an IQ test while you were in school. The tests are sometimes used to identify students who are struggling so they can be offered support. In fact, IQ tests were first developed in the beginning of the 20th century to identify students with learning problems. The questions were perhaps more entertaining: Students were asked to touch their noses or ears and draw a design from memory. Now IQ tests are very different.

IQ tests are also used for adults. An early use of IQ tests for adults was to select those with high scores for the armed forces. Today, medical examinations sometimes incorporate these tests to check whether a patient has good language skills. Employers can also use the tests as part of a job interview. Although very little evidence suggests that a good IQ score leads to a higher salary or makes someone a more productive employee; nonetheless, many employers still use the tests.

You can find a range of tests on the Internet that claim to give you an accurate score for your language skills. However, remember that online tests are rarely accurate, and they haven't undergone the strict scientific rigour of making sure that the tests measure your language skills in a reliable and valid manner. Don't worry though. If you're interested in finding out what your verbal IQ is, many tests are scientifically valid and can provide insight into your language skills.

## *Measuring your brain's verbal IQ*

Would you like to test your verbal IQ? Here are some examples of questions you can answer that can help you do so:

- ✔ How are a dog and a cat the same?
- ✔ How are an apple and an orange the same?

You may have guessed that this type of tests measures how well you can compare things in the world around you. You may have said that a dog and a cat are both animals, which is a good response. But a better response would be that they're both domesticated animals or pets. What about an apple and an orange? Some people point out that they're both round and, of course, they're both fruits. The purpose of this test is to measure how well you can verbalise how two different things (dog and cat) can be considered alike.

Try some different ones now:

- ✔ Give a short definition for the word *fashion*.
- ✔ Give a short definition for the word *democracy*.

The answers that you give for these questions tend to reflect your own experiences. For example, you may define *fashion* as 'useless' or 'a waste of time'. Although this may be an accurate reflection of your own views, you'll probably get a score of zero. A good answer would be 'a prevailing style or custom'. This answer would get a score of 2. An IQ test like this measures not only how well you know the definition of a word, but also how well you can verbalise this definition.

Try one more set of examples:

- ✔ What would you do if you saw someone running off with a bag and a woman crying 'Help'?
- ✔ What would you do if you saw someone struggling in the water?

These questions measure how well you can respond to social situations and apply your common sense. Here again, your experiences may direct your responses. For example, you may have just read in the news about a man who successfully chased away a burglar from his house and, inspired by this story, you respond that you'd stop the person running off with the bag. Related to the second question, you may have a fear of water and so you wouldn't want to jump in to help a struggling person.

Psychologists and statisticians have carefully vetted the questions in a verbal IQ to make sure that they provide an accurate measure of your language skills. After completing an IQ test, you get a score that can range between 50 to 150.

So what does your score mean? Most people get a score in the average range: between 85 to 115. That's pretty good. But some people get above average: a score of 130 or higher. Less than 3 per cent of the population get a score like this; it's very rare. On the flip side, some people get a low score, perhaps close to 50. Here again, a tiny percentage of the population gets such a score. But don't worry, scientific evidence shows that IQ actually plays a very small role in your life successes. In fact, your memory plays a big role, which is why keeping your brain healthy is so important.

# Chapter 7

# Recognising Faces and Remembering Directions

*In This Chapter*

▶ Boosting your visual and spatial skills

▶ Using easy tricks to keep your visual and spatial skills intact

▶ Testing your memory

**Y**ou're offered two apples. How do you choose between them? Chances are that you'll pick the bigger one; I would. But you may have also used colour or other visual features, such as whether there was a bruise on it, to choose between the two apples. Did you know that you're using your visual-spatial memory skills to make that decision? You kept the image of one apple in mind while looking at the other. Even the simplest everyday things require you to use your visual-spatial memory skills.

In this chapter I cover tips on how to develop your visual and spatial skills.

## Understanding Visual-Spatial Memory Skills

Visual-spatial memory skills are how you learn about the world, right from the beginning. As a baby, your visual-spatial skills are fantastic. Perhaps because babies haven't yet developed language skills, they're able to take a snapshot of the world and remember certain visual features. Think for a moment of the world of a baby. You present the baby with a toy. How does he know whether this toy is a new one that he hasn't seen before or an old toy from his toy box? He has to bring up his mental images of his toys and decide whether this new toy in front of him matches the images in his head. Psychologists suggest that babies remember the features of their toys and other aspects of the world around them: colour, shape, and specific features such as buttons for eyes, floppy ears, and so on.

What do babies and toys have to do with you as an adult? The process is not so different from what you do when you meet someone new. You may even think, 'He looks familiar. Have I met this person before?' Or you may be even more specific and look at his hair and think, 'He reminds me of Uncle Jack. He has the same hair colour.' These types of thoughts suggest that you're using your visual-spatial memory skills as an adult to learn about faces, much like babies do with toys.

# Banishing the 'You Look Familiar, But I Can't Remember You' Phenomenon

You know the feeling. You're at a social function, and a friend greets you and says, 'You remember Joe.' And you look at Joe and know that you should remember Joe – he does look familiar – but you just can't place him. Where do you know him from – work, the gym, the local café, your kids' school or sports?

If it makes you feel any better, the 'You look familiar, but I can't remember your name' phenomenon happens to everyone. As you get older, forgetting names is simply part of the aging process. The reason for this occurrence is the slow decay of some of the brain connections involved in this process.

## I only know you if you're famous

What's remarkable is that your memory for names of famous faces tends to be preserved. Psychologists have found that even healthy *elderly* people (defined as age 60 to 91) have great memories for famous faces and can even remember information about the famous people based on their faces. For example, when shown a photo of Celine Dion, these mature adults could identify that she was a singer and even name one or two of her songs.

Adults in the early stages of Alzheimer's disease struggle with placing the name when looking at a photo of a famous face. Their memory (or lack of it) for famous faces offers an important clue, and some psychologists suggest that memory for faces should be used as an early detection tool of Alzheimer's disease.

# You look like Joe!

Psychologists at Miami University have confirmed that people have a certain idea of what someone called Joe or Mary should look like. But what's more interesting is that the better a face matches a name, the more likely you are to remember the person.

The psychologists asked a group of people to create a series of faces using computer software. They then asked another group to rate how well they thought a name fitted a face. Finally, the psychologists asked a third group of people to remember the faces and the names. If the face was paired with a name that didn't 'fit' very well, then people found it hard to remember. People really do have an idea of what Joe and Mary should look like!

So the next time you have to remember someone's name, why not think of a name that 'fits' and make an association? Think of Ramon, who looks like a Joe, and remember the acronym RJ.

What happens if you can't afford to forget people's names? You can train your brain to remember those faces.

Psychologists have recently discovered that your brain still stores forgotten faces. You just need to know how to unlock the memories of the faces. Psychologists showed people pictures and then waited a while and showed them the same pictures again and asked the people if they'd seen the pictures before. When people could clearly remember what they saw, there was a strong brain wave pattern. However, when they were struggling to remember whether they'd seen the pictures previously, the same brain wave pattern existed; it just wasn't as strong. This means that your brain remembers when you've have seen something before even if you don't know it! Chapter 4 and 5 offers tips on how to train your brain to remember new information.

Even simple tasks like configuring the settings on a new phone require visual-spatial skills. You have to look at the manual, keep that information in mind and then transfer your focus to your phone. In contrast to language skills, you actually have a much smaller 'space' to remember visual-spatial information. Psychologists suggest that, on average, people can only remember three or four visual images. So don't feel too bad if you struggle to remember everyone's names at the office party or always stop to ask for directions.

## *Reasoning and logic: The key to training your visual-spatial skills*

The good news is that you can improve your visual-spatial skills. The first step is to test them. Try this fun example below.

### *Testing your logic and reasoning*

Figure 7-1 shows a common task that instructors give to psychology students to test their logic and reasoning skills. You see four cards, with only one side showing.

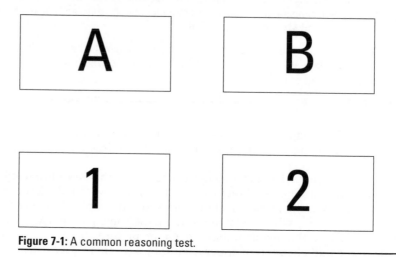

**Figure 7-1:** A common reasoning test.

Here's the rule: if one side of the card displays a vowel, then the other side of the card can only show an even number.

Which card do you turn over to check this rule? Most people turn over the card with the letter A. That's correct. Now which card do you turn over next? You may be tempted to turn over the card with the number 2. But this wouldn't be correct. You should turn over the card with the number 1.

Why? Look at the rule again: if one side of the card displays a vowel, then the other side of the card can only show an even number.

You turned over the card with the letter A to confirm this rule because A is a vowel. You don't need to turn over the card with letter B because the rule said nothing about consonants. When it comes to the card with the number 1, you may have thought that you don't need to turn this over. But you do need to check whether it has a vowel on the other side. If it does have a vowel, then it's violated the rule. You don't need to turn over the card with the number 2 because the rule doesn't state what should happen if you have an even number on one side.

If you're still puzzling over this, don't worry. Most people find this test very difficult. Try this version.

Here's the rule: if you're under 21, you can't drink alcohol.

You're the bartender and you have to make sure that no one breaks this rule. Figure 7-2 shows what you see at one table.

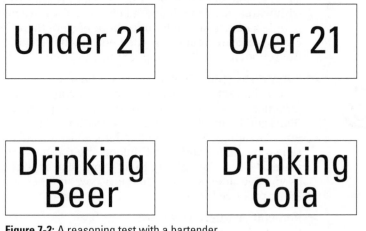

**Figure 7-2:** A reasoning test with a bartender.

Whose age will you check? You'll probably check the first person who's under 21. And you'd also check the person drinking beer to make sure that he's over 21. You aren't worried about the person drinking cola because it doesn't matter whether he's older or younger than 21 because cola isn't an alcoholic drink.

These kinds of tasks aren't meant to frustrate psychology students (though they may do that too!), but to illustrate how people use logic and reasoning in everyday situations. In the scenario with the drinks, you can save time by checking only certain people's ages, rather than checking everyone's age. In the later section 'Testing, testing' you can do a quick test of your skills.

### Using your reasoning skills to the max

Life presents you with many opportunities to recognise patterns and use your reasoning skills to their full potential.

Here are some suggestions that can help you strengthen the patterns and associations you may need daily:

- **Face facts.** Test your visual memory. Look at famous faces and see how fast you can come up with the people's names. Too easy? Try to come up with one fact about each person. Remember, don't just use 'celebrity' faces, but try to include political and historical figures as well.

- **Remember me.** Try the 'face facts' game with familiar faces. Start with people you know well – family members and close friends. This time, try to state five things you know about each person. Now look at photos of people you may not know as well – maybe colleagues from work or friends from school with whom you're no longer in contact. Try to remember the people's names and one thing about each of them. For the work colleague, remember the department he worked in; for the school friend, remember a funny incident that you shared.

- **Filter distractions.** You're more prone to forget things when you're distracted. So the next time someone's giving you directions over the phone, go somewhere quiet, shut the door, and focus only on the conversation. When you're introduced to someone new, look at him, shake his hand, and repeat his name, and stop thinking about refilling your empty plate or glass. Your ability to filter out distractions gets worse as you get older, so make an effort now so it becomes an automatic practice for you.

- **Remember where you were.** Your brain remembers odd little bits of information, such as the smell of the freshly cut grass in the park when your friend gave you directions to the party on the weekend, or the smell of the canapés at the office party as your boss introduced you to an important potential client. These bits of information that your brains stores may seem irrelevant, but they can serve as powerful clues to trigger your memory. When you're trying to remember something, think back to where you were when you first heard the information. Do you remember anything specific about the location? What was the person wearing? What were you doing? All these questions can help you reconstruct the moment, which in turn unlocks your memory.

- **Make your own box.** It's not for nothing that the saying 'Think outside the box' has caught on. People who can think beyond what others normally do have an advantage. They're more creative and come up with ideas that the others only talk about. If you can't find a solution right away, maybe you're approaching the problem in the wrong way. Try to ask different questions. The solution may surprise you.

# Working Your Memory Muscle

You store information in different parts of your brain. The brain keeps visual information in one part, and spatial information in another. However, your brain is very efficient in combining information from different parts to work together when you need to remember something.

The *hippocampus* is located in the temporal lobe of the brain and is responsible for storing spatial memory and helping you navigate. Individuals who suffer damage to their hippocampus also experience a negative effect of their spatial memory. This explains why these individuals feel disoriented and forget where they are or where they're going.

However, you can do a lot of things to keep your visual-spatial skills sharp and active. A study of nuns showed how their regular use of language preserved their brain functions even in old age. The same can be true for you.

In order to keep your visual-spatial skills sharp, here are some tips:

✔ **Puzzle me this.** Jigsaw puzzles aren't just for kids! They're a great way to boost your visual-spatial skills and develop your ability to see patterns. I love doing jigsaws and remember one family holiday where my dad and I stayed up all night to complete a particularly tricky puzzle. We were exhausted the next day but it was worth it!

An added bonus to that feeling of accomplishment is that jigsaw puzzles develop your visual-spatial memory skills. You have to recognise patterns between the pieces and learn to predict what you think the piece represents. This means that you have to keep in mind what the complete picture looks like and try to match the place of a single piece. People tend not to use these skills very often in everyday activities, so doing a puzzle is a great way to target these skills.

✔ **Spot the difference.** *Change blindness* is a term that psychologists use to describe people's inability to spot changes in scenes around them. In many experiments a man stops to ask for directions and halfway through, a woman takes the man's place. Most people don't even notice! A lot of newspapers and magazines include pictures where you have to spot the difference between two pictures. If you used to flip passed this puzzle, from now on take a moment to see how quickly you can do it.

## Drive a taxi!

A group of psychologists in London were interested in the brains of taxi drivers. In particular, they wanted to know whether their visual-spatial skills were better than other people's.

There are many reasons why their visual-spatial skills may be better than other people's. For starters, directions are taxi drivers' lifeblood – they need to know their way inside and out of a city like London. They also have to take an extensive test called the Knowledge, which requires drivers to know over 400 routes. The Knowledge is so demanding that 75 per cent of people drop out of the course. Yet fantastic gains exist for those who do stick with the course. Of course, a financial incentive exists – drivers stand to make significantly more money after passing the test.

However, a surprise bonus exists, as the psychologists discovered: taxi drivers have bigger brains! Yes, it's true. The part of brain associated with directions (visual-spatial memory) is actually larger in experienced taxi drivers compared to the average individual. The brain changes to accommodate the increasing amount of information on navigating and directions that taxi drivers have to take in.

This is an exciting study because it demonstrates that the brain has a certain amount of flexibility and can expand in response to certain information. Previously, psychologists found brain changes only in patients who'd sustained a brain injury, but in the case of the taxi drivers you see that everyone can benefit from working their memory muscles.

Use everyday situations to use your visual-spatial skills to spot the difference. When you walk into your supermarket, try to pick out three things that are different from the last time you were there. Are the vegetables in the same place? How about the eggs? Training your eyes to focus on things that are different not only makes you more observant, but also preserves these skills that you need to remember faces and directions.

# Looking at Visual-Spatial IQ Tests

Psychologists use a range of different tests to look at how the brain works and to measure visual-spatial ability, from looking at pattern sequences to recognising shapes, and even remembering faces. An important point to remember is that IQ tests go through many different rounds of checking to ensure that the test is an accurate measure of visual-spatial ability. Another key feature of standardised IQ tests is that the score you receive is based on data from thousands of people from the same age group as you, so your performance is being compared to your peer group.

In this section, I provide examples of tests that measure your visual-spatial ability.

## Testing, testing

The purpose of visual-spatial IQ tests is to measure your nonverbal (non-language) skills. Visual-spatial skills are one of the first abilities to develop, yet they decline much faster than language skills. Several reasons for this exist. One possibility is that people lose visual-spatial skills as a natural progression of aging. You forget names to faces, directions to places you've always walked or driven to, even when your holiday photos were taken.

As you get older, you take longer to come up with an answer because you have so many more life experiences so it takes longer to sift through them all to find the right word or image. So take heart: you take longer because you're wiser.

So how do you know when forgetting directions and faces is the result of being an extensive 'library' of wonderful and special life experiences and not the start of a downhill pattern? That's when IQ tests come in. They measure how well you use visual-spatial skills to understand patterns, recognise faces, and use logical reasoning. Most IQ tests ask you to complete a range of different activities and you can see examples of these in the next section.

You may have come across an IQ test while you were in school. The tests are sometimes used to identify students who are struggling so that they can be offered support. In fact, IQ tests were first developed in the beginning of the 20th century to identify students with learning problems. The questions were perhaps more entertaining: students were asked to touch their nose or ear and draw a design from memory. Now IQ tests are very different.

IQ tests are also used for adults. An early use of IQ tests for adults was to select those with high scores for the armed forces. Today, medical examinations sometimes incorporate these tests to check whether a patient has good visual-spatial skills, just as I explain in the earlier sidebar 'I only know you if you're famous' that how well you can recognise famous faces is a good indication of early signs of Alzheimer's disease.

Employers can also use the tests as part of a job interview, particularly tests that measure logical reasoning and pattern-matching skills. Something to remember though, is that IQ tests are different from tests that measure your job-specific skills, or knowledge that is specific to your job. IQ tests measure knowledge like the example in Figure 7-3. Very little evidence suggests that a good IQ score leads to a higher salary or makes someone a more productive employee.

You can find a range of tests on the Internet that claim to give you an accurate score for your visual-spatial skills. However, remember that it can be difficult to establish the accuracy of online tests, and they may not have undergone strict scientific rigour to make sure that the tests measure your visual-spatial skills in a reliable and valid manner. If you're interested in finding out what your nonverbal IQ is, many tests are scientifically valid and can provide insight into your visual-spatial skills.

## *Measuring your brain's visual-spatial IQ*

Would you like to test your visual-spatial IQ? Here are some examples of questions you can answer that can help you do so.

Take a look at Figure 7-3. Can you figure out the next shape in the sequence? You may have correctly guessed that the next shape will be a circle. As you are probably aware, this type of test measures how well you can spot the pattern and follow the sequence of objects. Other tests require you to construct a shape out of different coloured blocks. A key component in these tasks is that you gain extra points the faster you do these tasks.

**Figure 7-3:** A visual-spatial IQ test.

In timed tests, older people tend to lose points. However, when you remove the timed aspect, older people perform at the same level as younger people. But remember, as you get older you may take longer on these tasks because you may have adopted a more methodical approach to problem-solving.

Other tests measure your reasoning skills. Take a look at these statements:

Bird–Nest     ?–Kennel

Hammer–Nail     ?–Paintcan

The purpose of these questions is to measure how well you can make associations between two things. First look at the word pair of Bird–Nest. Now look at the next word pair with the missing word: ?–Kennel. Use the relationship between 'bird' and 'nest' to figure out the word that goes with 'kennel'. Now look at the next word pair: Hammer–Nail. Try to work out what you think their association is and then figure out the correct word to pair with 'paintcan'. The correct answer to the former is dog, and for the latter the correct answer is paintbrush.

## *Scoring your test*

The questions that are included in a standardised visual-spatial IQ test have been carefully vetted to make sure that they provide an accurate measure of your nonverbal skills. Like in a verbal IQ test (see Chapter 6), after completing a visual-spatial IQ test you get a score that can range between 50 and 150. So what does your score mean?

Most people get a score in the average range, which is between 85 to 115. That's pretty good. But some people get above average: a score of 130 or higher. Less than 3 per cent of the population get a score like this; it's very rare. On the flip side, some people get a low score, perhaps close to 50. Here again, a tiny percentage of the population gets such a score. Don't panic, though – scientific evidence shows that IQ actually plays a very small role in your life successes. In fact, your memory plays a big role, which is why keeping your brain healthy is so important.

# Part III
# Fostering a Happy, Healthy Mind

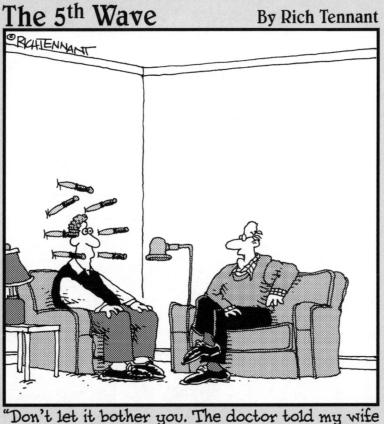

"Don't let it bother you. The doctor told my wife it would keep her mind sharp if she learned a new skill."

# In this part...

*A*re you a closet painter? Do you love to write? Or maybe you're one of those people who love singing in the shower? In this part you discover how you can use your passions and interests to train your brain. From activities to improve your creativity to spending a few minutes in meditation each day, you can try a range of ways that are proven to boost your brain's performance.

# Chapter 8

# Improving Your Creativity

From music to drawing, many ways exist to get your creative brain working. The benefits to getting your creative brain working include having the ability to 'think outside the box' at your workplace, come up with unique solutions to problems, and even to enjoy certain activities more.

Find something that you enjoy doing and make time to do the activity regularly. Your work life benefits from your creative activities as well.

In this chapter I talk about how to get your creative juices flowing.

## Boosting Your Brain Power with Creative Endeavours

Training your brain isn't all about hard work! *Creative thinking –* being able to come up with original solutions to problems – is a great way to encourage your brain to integrate information from different sources (see Chapter 2 for more on how the brain works). It means not giving up when a problem seems hard, but instead finding a different perspective – something unusual or unique.

Not everyone can become the next Beethoven or Da Vinci, but here are some suggestions of things that you can do to develop your creative side.

✔ **Be prepared.** 'Chance favours only the prepared mind.' This quote from a famous scientist (Louis Pasteur) sums up what scientists now know from studying brain patterns. Different parts of the brain show more activation just before a problem is presented. This means that the brain gets ready and gathers information from different parts in order to generate a solution.

When you're faced with a problem, the solution seldom comes from thin air. The answer is often the result of hours (and sometimes) years of preparation. So the next time you have a problem to tackle, do your homework and prepare well. A creative solution will soon follow.

✔ **Shh, no more talking.** Sometimes talking about a problem too much can ruin the creative process. Studies have found that the creative process works best if you're not constantly vocalising your plans. In many ways the creative solution is an automatic process. Some even suggest that creativity has a subconscious element to it – you're creative without even thinking about being creative. So the next time you're trying to be creative, avoid talking about it and let your brain do the work.

✔ **Look away.** Sometimes focusing on a problem for too long can reduce your creativity. Scientists have now found evidence that the brain produces an excessive amount of *gamma waves*, which is linked to excessive amounts of attention, when you focus on a problem for too long. This increase in gamma waves leads to a mental roadblock, which of course won't help you solve the problem. (See Chapter 10 to find out about brain waves and sleep.)

So if you've lost your creative vibe, it's time to get up and walk away from the problem. Do something else for a bit – anything else, as long as the activity isn't related to the problem you're trying to solve. Let your mind rest for a time so when you come back your brain is recharged.

Studies have found that people who use their creative skills for their work can end up struggling to balance their responsibilities at home and at work. Because the creative process isn't often confined to an office space, they often do work-related tasks outside of normal work hours. As a result, these people can experience more job pressure, which impacts social and family relationships.

If you're involved in a creative work environment, try to see the positive side of your job. Most creative people enjoy thinking about their work and coming up with creative solutions. Creative work isn't a stressful problem that they have to solve that can keep them awake at night. Instead, creative work gives people a sense of accomplishment and fulfilment, especially when they find a solution. Remember to focus on the satisfaction you get from using your creative skills, rather the potential stress of solving a problem (see Chapter 9 for more on managing stress and anxiety).

# Tapping Out Tempo

'If music be the food of love, play on.' Based on evidence of the power of music for the brain, I'd like to change this famous quote from the opening of *Twelfth Night* by Shakespeare to, 'If music be the food of the brain, play on.'

From infants to the elderly, music has a power over the brain. Music can make the brain think in more creative ways.

Here are some tips to help you encourage your musical side:

- ✔ **Sing along.** Infants respond to the pitch and rhythm of language. The term *motherese* refers to the high pitch, cooing voice that mothers (and fathers too, but the term *dadese* hasn't really caught on!) often use to speak to their babies. Studies demonstrate that babies pick up on these pitch patterns and coo back, following the same patterns. Early communication is characterised by mimicking the tempo and rhythm of language. When the mother coos in a certain way, the baby does too.

- ✔ **Play music to pay attention.** Music lessons help students learn to pick up on classroom instructions better. Research has found that playing an instrument is useful in helping youngsters filter out noisy distractions in the classroom and focus on the teacher's voice more accurately. Playing a musical instrument doesn't just teach the brain to turn up the volume of all sounds, but helps the brain to discriminate the noise from the relevant information effectively.

  When someone learns a musical instrument, she trains her brain to extract the relevant musical patterns, such as harmony and rhythm. The brain is then able to apply this same skill to filtering and picking up on language and other sounds, whether in the classroom or at the playground.

---

# Music for learning

Music can even help those with cochlear implants learn language faster. A *cochlear implant* is an electronic device that's surgically implanted to improve hearing. Some infants are born with hearing impairments that not even hearing aids can help. These babies receive a cochlear implantation procedure. Although the operation may be a success, the baby has never heard speech before and must learn to understand language. Research has found that music therapy is tremendously beneficial in helping previously deaf children learn to communicate. These children are able to follow the rhythm and pitch of language much better, which eventually increases the speed at which they learn to talk.

---

- ✔ **Listen to the sound of music.** Listening to music activates different parts of the brain related to attention, memory, and processing information and emotions. What's really powerful is that music can heal the adult brain as well. Studies reveal that just listening to music can result in faster cognitive recovery in stroke patients. The patients' verbal memory and attention improves faster compared to people who just listen to audio books. As a bonus, listening to music during stroke recovery also prevents negative moods, such as depression.

- ✔ **Improve your memory.** Studies found that when you put words to music, the memory of people with Alzheimer's improves significantly. Parts of the brain associated with memory (see Chapter 2) work at a slower pace in those with Alzheimer's disease. However, putting words that you need to remember to music creates a stronger memory link than just repeating the words on their own. So if you know someone with Alzheimer's disease who's struggling to remember daily tasks, put the list of jobs to music and sing the list to the person.

## Music and language development

Baby talk is often very musical and fathers, mothers, grandparents, and even strangers seem to take on this way of speaking naturally when talking to a baby. Common features of their speech include speaking in a rhythmic manner, with up-and-down sing-song tones and high pitches. Of course, every parent wants to know if using baby-talk will help her child learn to speak faster. Before I answer this question, it's important to know that two types of baby-talk exist:

✔ The most common form features a slower cadence, the use of a high-pitched voice, frequent repetition, and simplifying sentences.

✔ The second type of baby-talk includes all the features of the previous bullet point, as well as made-up words such as *wa-wa* and *din-din*.

The first kind of baby-talk is very important to language learning. Research has found that the high-pitched voice can help a child discover the structure of language. For example, you use rising intonation to mark the end of a sentence. Furthermore, vocal stress on verbs helps to draw the baby's focus to important information in a sentence. Also, when parents use short words and frequent repetition they direct the child to key objects or events in her environment. This uncomplicated structure of speaking can be useful in helping your baby pick up grammatical rules.

Baby-talk also has an important function in a baby's social development. The one-to-one interaction aids a child's social integration because the high-pitched voice lets the child know that the mother is specifically addressing her, helping her prepare for more complex exchanges. Your baby can use baby-talk to pick up vocal cues to determine turn-taking in conversation. For example, the rising intonation in the mother's voice is a signal to the child that her turn is ending and it's time for the child to begin her turn. This provides an opportunity for the baby to learn to engage in the give and take of conversation.

The second type of baby talk can actually do more harm than good. You may be surprised to know that if you use made-up words you could delay your child's speech development. Babies imitate their parent's speech, and if you constantly use nonsensical words during this critical period in your child's language development then she's learning words that have no relevance in real-life situations. As she grows older, the child's conversations with peers is peppered with nonsense words, leaving the child at a disadvantage. Furthermore, research has shown that children develop best with speech that challenges them by being more complex than their own. So, if you've been using a great many nonsense words when you speak with your baby, try to speak to her using everyday vocabulary instead.

Scientific research confirms that the musical nature of baby talk helps a baby to develop language. Communication is like a game of tennis, with pauses for the listener to jump in with a comment. Baby talk is a tool to show a baby that language is interactive, and not just a list of commands.

Although listening to music can help develop memory and language skills in children, keep in mind that no substitute exists for spending time with your child. Many DVDs promote the idea of the *Mozart effect* – that listening to Mozart makes your child smarter (see Chapter 3 for more about this topic). But if you really want to see the full benefits of music, get involved with your child. Sing to your child, clap with her, make up songs together, teach her how to play a musical instrument. All these activities harness the power of music for your child's brain much more than simply putting in a DVD and sitting her down in front of it.

If you're one of those people who think that your singing should never leave the shower because you can't carry a tune, you're not alone. Around 10 per cent of the population is *tone deaf* – which means that they can't sing in tune. Tone-deaf people also can't consciously tell that their singing is off-key. New scientific research has identified a specific brain circuit that links sound perception with producing language that's missing in people who are tone deaf. It may be that tone deafness is an early sign of a language disorder.

## Perfecting your pitch to keep your brain

Scientific evidence demonstrates that musical training improves memory – musicians tend to remember more information compared to non-musicians, even when you take their education levels and their ages into account. In other words, playing a musical instrument activates part of the brain (the cerebral cortex), which in turn boosts recall of information.

Music training is good for school work. When children are exposed to music lessons that involve complex rhythms and tones, they usually have better reading skills compared to children of the same age who don't have music lessons. But it's not just reading that improves. Psychologists have found that maths skills and spatial reasoning are also better in students who receive music lessons (see Chapter 7 for examples of spatial reasoning tasks).

What is it about music that helps children use their brain better in school? When people hear music, it activates different systems across the brain. In addition to working memory (see the sidebar 'Does practice really make perfect?' in this chapter), the brain also processes musical information using both the left and right hemispheres of the brain (see Chapter 2 for an inside look at the brain). This use of different parts of the brain during musical instruction can also impact how children learn.

# Does practice really make perfect?

I remember my piano lessons when I was growing up. My teacher was old school and used to sit next to me with a ruler while I played. Every time my hands drooped on the keyboard, I'd get a sharp rap on the knuckles! The teacher was very strict and I had to practise every day.

Despite this strict teaching, I do love playing the piano and still play today. But did all my practising lead me to become a musical genius? Sadly, no. The only time I enter a concert hall is as a member of the audience. Maybe I should have practised more!

People debate whether musical genius is inherited (you're born with it) or whether someone can practise to achieve this level of expertise. The current view is that is takes years of intense practice to become an expert.

But it's not just practice that makes the difference. *Working memory* – the ability to keep information in mind and manipulate it – is crucial in musical skills as well. For example, pianists use working memory when they read music. For example, they are usually looking ahead to read the notes that are coming next. This is a skill that most expert musicians have.

Psychologists asked a group of expert pianists to sight-read a selection of musical sheets. So how could the pianists play a song from a music sheet that they'd never seen before? Of course, practice was important. But also important were the pianists' working memory skills. Expert musicians need to have good working memory in order to achieve the next level of expertise. Without good working memory, they can only experience a limited level of success.

But *when* you teach music is as important as *what* to teach. Studies have found that growth spurts in brain development occur up until the age of 7. So simply saying that music makes you smarter isn't accurate. If you're going to provide music lessons, introduce the lessons by 7 years of age, if not before then, if you want to also see benefits in reading, maths, and reasoning skills.

If you're too embarrassed to sing karaoke with friends, you can use music in other ways to boost your brain. Here are some things that you can try:

✔ **Clap your hands.** It sounds surprising but children who sing songs that involve hand clapping have better skills, like neater handwriting and fewer spelling mistakes. It may be that the motor skill component of hand clapping helps in the classroom too. Because kids tend to love clapping while they're singing, it's a great opportunity to develop the motor component part of the brain. But clapping isn't just for kids' songs.

Make an effort to clap along when you hear a song. Focus on the beat of the song and clap in tempo. This trains your brain to follow the tempo.

✔ **Get a drum.** Rhythm links to working memory skills. For example, something as simple as being able to remember the sequence of taps relates to how well you can remember what someone's just told you. Most information involves a sequence. For example, you have to remember things in the order that you were told. This progression of doing one thing first, then another, then the next and finally the last is very similar to how people remember a sequence of sounds. So the next time you listen to a song, pay attention to the beat to boost your memory (see Chapter 19 for ideas on brain games that you can play on the move).

✔ **Write a song.** You don't have to be Beethoven or Beyoncé to come up with a song. Remember when you were a kid and loved to make up silly songs? My little boy comes up with all sorts of funny words and we sit at the piano together and come up with a song for the words.

As an adult, you can keep your love of singing and making music alive. The easiest place to start is with a sentence that expresses your emotions. Write a few lines and then put a little tune to the lines. If you can't come up with a tune on your own, why not use one from a song you like? The goal of this activity is to integrate different parts of the brain during song writing – from writing words to thinking of the music and the tempo, and putting it all together. Who knows, you may even get your family to start singing your songs!

Many benefits of listening to music exist, from improving language skills to recovering faster from a stroke. However, if you're trying to concentrate, listening to music (and singing along!) can distract you. Studies have found that when people do two things at the same time, they become less efficient and make more mistakes. And it doesn't make any difference whether you enjoy the music you're listening to or not – having music on can still cause you to make more mistakes. In one study researchers asked people to remember a list of words and do some mental maths tasks while listening to music they liked; listening to music they didn't like; or in quiet environment. People did the best on the tasks when they did them in a quiet environment. So although music is great for your brain, it's not so good if you're listening to it while doing something that demands your attention. If you're a music lover, instead of playing tunes in the background, why not enjoy your music beforehand and then get started on what you need to do? Which reminds me . . . hang on while I turn off the radio!

## Music at any age

If you close your eyes and listen to Jackie Evancho sing, you'll be immediately transported to an elegant opera hall with beautiful stage sets and a talented orchestra. Standing in the centre of the stage, you might imagine Jackie to be an elegant woman with years of opera training that have given her this voice of an angel that you now hear floating through the air. You might imagine her standing with her arms outstretched, reaching to you as she sings with a passion and a depth drawing from years of experience.

When you open your eyes, nothing could be farther from that image. Jackie isn't an elegant woman with years of training and experience. Jackie isn't a woman at all! She's a 10-year-old girl who only started singing two years ago, who's released an album and is the youngest female vocal soloist to have performed at Carnegie Hall in New York.

For Jackie, singing began after she went to watch *Phantom of the Opera* when she was 8 years old. She couldn't stop singing the songs. With the help of a voice coach, she's now made multiple TV appearances and over 3 million people have watched her sing! So if you feel like being inspired, look Jackie up – you won't be disappointed.

Which part of the brain is involved in processing music? The right hemisphere is more involved in processing pitch, melody, and harmony, as well as structure and meaning in musical sequences (see Chapter 2 for more on the brain functions). But is processing music a skill that all people are born with, or does someone develop the ability as a result of musical training? Studies using brain imaging to measure brain activity of newborns (those who were just a few days old) found that the infant brain already comes equipped with specific and specialised functions for understanding music. The right hemisphere processes Western music that's *tonal* (in other words, it has varying pitches). However, the left hemisphere (the left inferior frontal cortex) processes music that's *dissonant* (or not harmonious).

# Drawing Isn't Just for Picasso

If you've never thought of yourself as a creative person, it's time for a change of thinking. Each person has the potential to unlock an aspect of creativity. In the following section I list a few suggestions to help you get going. I've included tips on simple drawing activities to get you started, but if you feel that you still need more encouragement, why not simply begin by doodling?

## Doodling to stay on task

Are you a doodler? Do you find your papers covered in scribbles and scrawls? Well, now scientific research supports your efforts to stave off boredom. A recent study compared the working memory of two groups of people: doodlers and non-doodlers. Both groups were asked to listen to a pre-recorded phone message about a birthday party and asked to remember the names of the people coming. The doodling group remembered more names and places mentioned in the phone message compared to the non-doodlers. Doodling while listening can be beneficial because it helps the individual focus and maintain attention instead of tuning out altogether. Doodling isn't a demanding activity, and it acts like a buffer that prevents other activities like daydreaming from interfering with what you have to remember. So if you're worried that you'll start zoning out during a meeting, grab a pencil!

## Drawing to release your creative side

Drawing increases your imagination, which is critical in helping you find creative solutions to problems. So if doodling is like child's play to you, and you feel you're capable of drawing something a little more demanding than squiggles on the page, go ahead and dive right in.

Here are some ideas to get you drawing and unleashing your creative side:

- ✔ **Make a maze.** Start with one thought. It doesn't have to be profound; it can even be an object if that's easier. Write down the thought on an A4 sheet of paper. Now think of another thought. How can you connect the two ideas? Keep going until your paper looks like a maze of thoughts and ideas. The maze may not make sense in the beginning. But after a few tries, you'll find that this process becomes easier. And you'll notice that your brain starts making connections between different events more, which can start snowballing your creative process (see the section, 'Comparing the brains of creative and non-creative people', later in this chapter, for more on how the brain of a creative person works).

- ✔ **Make a card.** The next time you have to buy a card for someone's birthday, why not make one? Unlimited options for what you can do exist, from drawing a picture, to painting something, to even using old photos to recreate a precious memory you shared together. Not only is this a more meaningful way to share your thoughts, but making a card also lets you be creative.

## Rome was built in a day

Well, maybe not, but it was at least drawn in just two days. After a single 30-minute helicopter ride above the city in 2005, Stephen Wiltshire recreated the city from memory in amazing detail. Stephen is an architectural artist who draws and paints cityscapes from memory after just seeing them briefly. He was diagnosed with autistic spectrum disorder when he was a child and seemed to only enjoy drawing.

Stephen has a rare gift. He can draw a landscape after seeing it just once. For example, after flying over London in a helicopter, he was able to draw from memory a perfectly scaled aerial illustration of the area in just three hours. His drawing included over ten major landmarks and 200 buildings!

Stephen has drawn panoramic perspectives of cities all over the world: Sydney, Frankfurt, Madrid, Tokyo, Hong Kong, and New York have all been captured by his unique skill and mastery. His artworks are internationally recognised and recently broke auction records.

If making cards isn't something you like to do, then consider scrapbooking. You can finally do something with all those photos you have lying around and it's a great way to capture your memories. If most of your photos are digital, many online sites let you do virtual scrapbooking and share your pages with family and friends. (Read Chapter 11 for more on how socialising benefits your brain.)

✔ **Draw a cartoon.** Cartoons or even graphic novels are a great way to journal your thoughts. Instead of trying to find the right words to express how you felt today, why not draw a picture? You may even surprise yourself! If you feel brave, you can post your cartoons online using a blog and get your friends' feedback. You can also keep cartooning as something you do just for yourself. Whatever you choose, creating this type of diary is a fun way to express your thoughts and release a more creative you!

# Comparing the Brains of Creative and Non-creative People

To answer the question, 'is the brain of a creative person different from a non-creative person?' researchers looked at the brain activity of those who solve problems with that burst of 'Aha!' compared to those who solve problems more systematically. They asked participants to relax for a few minutes while they used *electroencephalograms* (EEGs) to record the electrical activity in their brains.

Next, they gave the participants an anagram to solve. Try one for yourself: MPXAELE (it spells EXAMPLE).

The brain activation patterns of the creative types and the methodical types were very different. Creative people use the right hemisphere of their brain when they're problem solving. Even when creative people aren't trying to figure out a solution to something, the right hemispheres of their brains are working. This pattern reveals that even daydreams and 'meaningless' thoughts of creative people are filled with different ideas.

An interesting pattern is that creative people are very flexible in their thinking. Think of a maze that has multiple paths that lead to other paths that link to new ones and so on. That's what the brain activity of the creative person is like. The creative person draws on different triggers that spark one thought that leads to another. For example, a conversation may trigger a picture the person saw last month, which sparks a thought she had last week, which leads her to a new idea.

The brain of a methodical thinker is different. It's like a straight road that starts at one end with the problem and moves systematically along a single path until it finds a solution. Methodical thinkers don't allow their brains to get distracted by other ideas, but just focus exclusively on what they need to do and the steps they'll take to solve the problem.

# Chapter 9

# Developing a Positive Mindset

**D**o you sometimes feel that life would be so much better if only you won the lottery? That happiness would be within your grasp if only . . . you fill in the blank. In this chapter I talk about how important it is to keep a positive outlook on life's bumpy road.

Sometimes, life can suddenly 'drop you in it', or 'throw you a curveball'. Just when you aren't expecting it, a crisis or problem can suddenly arise. Yet you have the power to determine how troubles affect you. If you let problems overwhelm you, that can lead to stress and anxiety and even impact how well your brain functions. If you choose to overcome issues, then you experience amazing benefits for your brain.

## Smiling Your Way to a Better Brain

'Smile and you'll find someone else smiling back at you.' I remember this little platitude – something on a card that a friend at school had given me – from growing up. As a young girl I liked the idea of having another face smiling back at me. But although a smile can make you feel good, you may be wondering whether it's really good for your brain.

Research shows that positive emotions like happiness and enjoyment are closely linked to good physical and mental health. In contrast, negative emotions like worry and sadness can worsen health. Even in countries where people struggle to meet their basic needs, such as a place to live and food to eat, positive emotions still boost health — all the more reason to look at the bright side of things in life!

## When everyday life has you stressed out

Major life events can trigger stress, but so can an accumulation of daily responsibilities that may feel overwhelming. When you have a growing number of things that demand your attention, you can easily feel stressed out. But instead of feeling overwhelmed, by adopting the right approach you can turn a potentially stressful situation into something positive in many ways. Here are some ideas:

✔ **Ask a question.** Instead of saying to yourself 'I can't do this' or 'It's too difficult for me', try re-phrasing as a question. Ask yourself 'How can I do this?' or 'How can I achieve this?' By giving yourself questions instead of negative statements, you can change the way you think to start imagining possibilities instead of seeing hurdles.

For example, if you're asked to complete a difficult project at work, don't let yourself feel overwhelmed by the prospect of what you have to accomplish. Instead, break your task down into smaller, more achievable goals that are guided by questions, What should I do first? How can I achieve this first step?, and so on.

✔ **Turn negative into positive.** Don't be too quick to see a situation as something negative. For example, maybe you didn't get that promotion at work, but find something positive. Could you use the extra time to spend more quality time with your family or embark on a project that you always wanted to do but didn't have the time? You may not always find it easy to focus on the silver lining of an unexpected situation, but try to think of something positive that can come out of a difficulty.

✔ **Have a hero.** Think of someone inspiring who's overcome a difficult situation to triumph in something. For example, Lance Armstrong was diagnosed with cancer, but he didn't let that stop him. He went on to win the Tour de France for several years in a row. He's the only person to win seven times, even breaking previous records along the way! Inspirational stories like Lance Armstrong's are fantastic because they can motivate people to create their own success stories that they can share with others.

EXAMPLE

# Believing in a dream

This is the story of a man who had a dream; a man who wanted to make kids' dreams come true too. He wanted to achieve his dream using a gift he believed that he had – drawing and art. Despite this wonderful and noble goal, this man encountered many difficulties in making his dream a reality. His first attempt at achieving this goal resulted in failure – the company that he set up with a friend collapsed. His second attempt was also disastrous, and he had to file for bankruptcy.

The third attempt saw a little more success. He managed to create a character that kids seemed to like – a funny little rabbit called Oswald. But shortly afterwards, for various legal reasons, he lost the rights to that character. You might think that by now the man would've just given up, and maybe started looking for a desk job instead of pursuing his dreams to draw and bring wonderful characters to life. But not this man. He wasn't going to let a few bumps along the way derail his dream.

It took 13 long, hard years before he saw any success from his efforts, but throughout this period he kept on trying. His next character was one that's endured – a little mouse called Mickey. Shortly afterwards, the man went on to produce full-length movies full of animated characters that children all over the world love – *Snow White and the Seven Dwarfs*, *Peter Pan* and *Alice in Wonderland* are some examples.

You may have guessed by now who I'm talking about – Walt Disney, a man who refused to be limited by his failures. The Walt Disney Company now owns multiple theme parts, as well as motion picture studios, record labels, TV cable networks, and hotels. All because one man wasn't going to allow a few setbacks dampen his dream.

## *Thinking positive*

What you read can have a greater impact on your brain than you think. Studies have found that even reading words that make you think of laughing are enough to change the way you behave. Even when people try to suppress what they're feeling, happy emotions seep through. So if you're wondering why you haven't got a skip in your step, check out your reading material. It may be time to swap the weepy stories for something more upbeat.

Try the following techniques to reap the benefits of positive thinking and optimism:

✔ **Never give up.** At one point or another, everyone stumbles along the way – whether with a start-up company that fails or a project that doesn't turn out as you'd hoped. The key is what you do after a setback. Do you feel sorry for yourself and avoid trying again? Or do you pick yourself back up and try again? Think of Walt Disney's story (see the nearby side-bar 'Believing in a dream') and similar inspirational stories. Keep reminding yourself that life isn't about the golden road to success; it's about the bumpy road of ups and downs and whether you're going to pick yourself up and move on.

✔ **Bye-bye stress.** Positive thinkers experience less stress than those who have more negative thoughts. People who have positive thoughts believe in themselves and what they can accomplish. This means that when something does go wrong, they look at how to turn the situation into some good and quickly find ways to overcome their setbacks. The result is that their positive outlook leads to less stress and anxiety, which means better mental health. So if you're a negative thinker, read the section 'Changing Perspectives', later in this chapter.

Lower stress levels lead to better mental health (see the upcoming section 'Taking stock of your brain's health').

# Learned helplessness

The scene was a college classroom. Students were subjected to increasingly loud and annoying noises that they could neither predict nor control. For an extended period of time, these noises punctuated the classroom and the students just had to sit there while the noises were playing. Nothing they did would make the noises stop.

A short time after the noise did eventually stop, the students were given a series of puzzles (anagrams) to solve. Most of the students really struggled, even though the classroom was now quiet. You might think that maybe the puzzles were just too difficult for them. But that wasn't the case. Another group of students who hadn't been exposed to the loud and unpredictable noises had no difficulty solving the puzzles at all.

Were the noises linked to how well the group who heard the noises could solve the puzzles? It appeared so. Even though the noises weren't played during the puzzle-solving time, the students felt helpless to control their situation – they couldn't make the noises stop. This sense of powerlessness affected their ability to perform in other tasks that had nothing to do with the noises.

The feeling of powerlessness to change your circumstance is known as *learned helplessness*. Some sports commentators use this term to describe a losing streak in a team – a series of losses results in a lack of control over events, which creates further losses. Could the opposite be true – a winning streak leads to a false sense of security? If the team you support lost that critical match, you might certainly think so. How else could they have lost!?

Learned helplessness can affect your view of life's events. If you feel that you can't control the events in your life, this can lead to passive acceptance of your circumstances and unwillingness to do anything to try to change anything. Eventually, this sense of lack of control can lead to depression.

# Changing Perspectives

You know the feeling – something isn't quite right and you can't stop thinking about it. *Rumination* is the term psychologists use to describe the process of trying to work things out in your head. Psychologists identify two types of rumination:

- ✔ **Reflection** is a positive response to a problem and can lead to finding a solution. This is when you consider the problem and come up with a plan of action to solve the problem.

- ✔ **Brooding** is more negative and is linked with strong emotions like worry and even fear. Brooding is when you replay something over and over in your head, or with a willing (or even unwilling!) listener. This type of behaviour usually results in stress because you're only focusing on the negative aspects of the situation ('poor me' syndrome), thinking about what you wished you'd said at that moment, for example, instead of actually thinking ahead and planning how to be proactive and solve the problem.

Slipping into a brooding mood can be easy when you keep replaying a scene or event in your head and when you're being self-critical, so don't do it! Sometimes you can be your own worst critic. Criticising yourself regularly can be damaging to your mental health and lead to a *self-fulfilling prophecy*, where you start believing what you think about yourself (for example, that you're a failure). The next time you feel like criticising yourself, stop and think about what you did right in that situation. List all the positive ways in which you responded. Try to come up with at least one thing, maybe even something as small as a smile. Focus on the positive things the next time your inner critic rises to point the finger at everything you did wrong.

Obsessively ruminating about something doesn't just steal away time, but also it can lead to more serious mental health problems. If you find yourself constantly worrying about something, take the following steps now to prevent yourself from slipping down a slope of negativity.

- ✔ **Keep your eye on the goal.** The goal is to resolve the problem. Don't let your mind wander and start feeling discouraged with statements like 'Things never work out for me'. These thoughts are unhelpful and won't help you reach a resolution. Write down what the problem is. Next, list two or three actions that you can carry out to solve the problem. Seeing the problem (and possible solutions) in writing makes a big difference and can stop brooding thoughts from swirling aimlessly around your mind. Be strict with yourself – if you notice that you start feeling sorry for yourself, read over the problem and start planning a solution.

✔ **Find a middle ground.** Sometimes you may need to lower expectations. Getting the perfect answer may not be possible. Don't get hung up; move on to find out the next best solution. Remember, a healthy brain is one that's free of brooding thoughts. So don't waste your mental energy wishing you could change the past. You can change your future circumstances by finding a workable solution.

✔ **Take time out.** Sometimes you need to take a break from the problem. Mentally walk away for a while. Maybe meet up with a friend and do something enjoyable together. Make a pact not to mention the problem at all during your time together.

✔ **Enlist a friend.** Asking for help isn't a sign of weakness. Don't carry the mental burden of a problem on your own. If you can't find the strength to come up with an action plan to address your problem, ask a friend to help you. If your problem is more serious, you may need to consider seeing a professional counsellor. Find one that's recommended and has good credentials.

Here's an example of how you can use these steps to resolve a problem. Perhaps you've decided to clear some financial debts. First, write down the amount that you'd like to pay off, and then identify two or three clear ideas of ways in which you plan to do this. Maybe you'll have to sacrifice some expensive dinners out with friends to put aside this money and pay off the debts. Remember to be realistic: obviously you need to eat, but ask yourself if you can eat on a smaller budget.

If you find yourself overwhelmed by the task of sorting through your finances, take a break. Call a friend and meet up. Just remember to pick an activity that doesn't cost a lot of money! Finally, it helps to be accountable, so tell a friend what you're trying to accomplish. This way, your friend can provide you with support when you say 'no' to certain social events.

## *Taking stock of your brain's health*

Apathy and depression can lead to 'cognitive impairment' (such as memory difficulties), which is a risk factor for Alzheimer's disease and dementia. Be aware of triggers that can lead your brain down a path of mental sadness and anxiety. Here are some issues that you should be aware of:

✔ **Avoiding the bottle.** If you're a man, beware of the bottle when you're stressed. Studies have found that, compared to women, men are more likely to drink alcohol after they've experienced a stressful situation. Men tend to use alcohol as a distraction to avoid confronting the stress. If drinking becomes a pattern, it could lead to alcohol abuse (see Chapter 13 for more on alcohol and your brain).

✔ **Looking away from the situation.** Women tend to focus on the negative aspects of a stressful situation – they ruminate or play over a scene again and again. As a result, women are more likely than men to say that they feel sad or anxious, which may lead to a higher risk of depression and anxiety disorders.

✔ **A place to call home.** Where you live makes a difference to your mental health. For example, women who live in crowded homes are more likely to be depressed than men. Why are more women affected by crowded living spaces than men? One explanation is down to how the sexes cope with stress (see the section 'Taking control to de-stress' in this chapter). Because women are more likely to adopt a 'tend and befriend' response, they gravitate toward social relationships to deal with stress. However, living in a crowded space means that their 'escape' involves social situations within that same physical environment. As a result, women can feel trapped in their environment without a change of scene.

The risks of developing Alzheimer's disease differ between men and women. You may be wondering what this has to do with your brain's health. If you're a woman then your mental health has a lot to do with whether you'll be affected by Alzheimer's disease. Studies have found that women who struggle to perform routine daily tasks because of clinical depression are more likely to progress to getting Alzheimer's disease. For women, depression is a greater risk factor than stroke (stroke is a risk factor for men). So take stock of your mental health early, especially if you're a woman.

Women are more likely than men to experience clinical depression and other anxiety disorders. Researchers suggest that this is because the female brain may not release the necessary hormones to allow the brain to adapt to stressful situations (see the 'Managing Stress and Anxiety' section in this chapter). So if you're a woman, you don't want stress to build up and overwhelm you. Take extra care to allow yourself time to unwind and relax.

## Why 'half-empty' doesn't make a difference to your mental health

You may be the type of person who sees the glass as half-empty instead of half-full. For example, if you were overlooked for a promotion at work, you may see it as as 'nothing good ever happens to me' – a sure sign of pessimism. Although everyone has days when things don't seem as bright as they could be, a *pessimist* is someone who sees things as worse than they really are and struggles to find solutions to problems. The result of pessimism is considerable stress, which can begin to wear away at mental health. However, being pessimistic is more than just seeing the glass as half-empty – it's an underlying sense of negativity that impacts not only how a person views himself, but also how he interprets events in his life.

But my research has found that your personality isn't an excuse for negative thoughts. In fact, *working memory* (the ability to remember and mentally process information) is much more important (see Chapter 5 for more information). As part of my own research, I studied 1,200 people aged from their late teens to their sixties, giving them a series of psychological tests and questionnaires. The results showed that people who have a high working memory tend to be more optimistic, more hopeful about life, more confident that they can cope with problems, more able to adjust to situations, and more likely to expect the best possible outcome from a situation. This finding is important because substantial evidence exists that people with a high sense of optimism are less likely to suffer serious illness. On the occasions when they do fall ill, their illnesses are less severe and they're better able to cope with their condition, and as a result recover faster.

People with a poor working memory spend more time brooding and get fixated on problems when they arise. These people often have a poor coping style in a time of crisis and instead of facing their problems straight on, they often abandon their goals instead. People who are 'brooders' are more likely to experience depression. They tend to focus on the negative aspects of a situation, which affects their mental health and increases their stress levels.

So what's the take-home message from all this? That a high working memory prevents you from fixating on a problem and allows you to be proactive in planning ahead to solve a problem.

# Managing Stress and Anxiety

Stress plays a major role in the development of several major mental health illnesses, including depression. One question that's of interest is why some people are more affected by stress than others. The answer may link to the *fight or flight* mechanism. When someone's faced with a stressful situation, does he avoid it (*flight*) or try to adapt and deal with it (*fight/cope*)? How you answer this question seems to offer a clue as to whether or not stress overwhelms you.

In a study of mice researchers found that those who avoided a stressful situation with larger, aggressive mice were more likely to experience stress. In contrast, those mice who found a way of adapting and coping with their situation had healthier brains. So the flight option isn't always the best. Sometimes working out how to adjust and cope is actually the less stressful alternative and is better for your mental health in the long term.

## Understanding why stress kills brain cells

What part of the brain is most affected by stress? Scientists have found that the hippocampus – which is linked to long-term knowledge and spatial memory (see Chapter 2) – suffers the most. This can explain why depression affects memory as well. A depressed person can also find it difficult to absorb new information (which is something the hippocampus is responsible for).

 Stress can also physically shrink your brain. Studies have found that high levels of stress can reduce the volume of the hippocampus, as well as the anterior cingulate cortex, which is linked to controlling stress hormones.

Stress kills – that's what people say. But is that statement really true? Well, yes and no. Some stress is good for your brain, but other types of stress aren't.

 Here are some top reasons to avoid stress in your life if you want your brain to be at its best:

✔ **Avoiding self-sabotaging behaviour.** Be aware of when your behaviours may be letting you down. In a stressful situation some people can respond in ways that can actually make the situation worse. Aggressive behaviour is one example. Asserting your feelings about a situation calmly without shouting or getting stressed out is better than being aggressive. Being assertive means that you state your point without bullying or manipulating someone else. You make your intentions clear in a calm manner. Other examples of self-sabotaging behaviour include overeating or overspending, instead of finding a healthy way to address the situation.

# The man who won too much

In what could possibly be described as the best investment ever, a man who we'll call Frank turned $7 into $27 million (and no, that's not a typo!), all in one day. How did he do it? By winning the lottery.

When people talk of happiness, the conversation inevitably leads to lottery winners. Most people think that winning the lottery is a way of escaping their present situation; that winning is going to lead to a better life, more opportunities, and certainly the big *H* – happiness.

But case after case reveals that money just doesn't buy happiness. In Frank's situation, he burned through his money in less than five years. Between millionaire-dollar homes, private jet hire and expensive trinkets, Frank was described as a sucker for 'deals' – he had so much money he just didn't know what to do with it and ended up buying the first shiny thing that caught his eye. Sadly, drugs were something else that caught his eye as well.

Today, Frank doesn't work and lives in a storage unit, having auctioned off his expensive cars and homes. This is hardly the life of someone who could have lived off almost $3 million a year for the next 25 years!

What happened with Frank and why do so many lottery winners end up unhappier than before they won? For starters, the brain stops registering the lottery win as an amazing event. This feeling is described as *habituation* – where you get used to what you have. After a while the buzz wears off and all the winner is left with is bits of printed paper that he didn't work for and doesn't know how to spend.

Things in life that are more important, such as family and relationships, can get shelved in exchange for hoarding the money, which can contribute to a feeling of unhappiness. Ultimately, it seems that the old saying that 'Money can't buy happiness' is true, certainly for lottery winners.

✔ **Dropping the blood pressure.** Stress leads to hypertension and high blood pressure. In a group of almost 1,000 adults aged 65 years and older, scientists found that those with high blood pressure were at a greater risk of mild cognitive impairment. This means that these adults found it harder to focus, had a hard time performing simple cognitive activities and reported that they forgot things more frequently.

✔ **Slipping down the slope.** If you think that a little forgetfulness is something that you can live with, think again. Mild cognitive impairment can lead to dementia and Alzheimer's disease (see Chapters 6 and 7). As much as 15 per cent of people who experience mild cognitive impairment subsequently struggle with dementia and Alzheimer's. Studies have found that mild cognitive impairment is the most robust predictor for memory-loss disease; in other words, educational level, whether you're male or female and where you live are much less important. So making sure that your stress levels don't hit the roof is all the more important. Yet another reason to make sure that you spend your weekends relaxing rather than working!

# *Taking control to de-stress*

Men and women respond to stress differently. While men tend to adopt the fight or flight response, women are more likely to adopt a *tend and befriend* response. This means that women respond by nurturing others (the tend response) and joining forces with other people so they have a support group in the time of stress (the befriend response).

Brain imaging studies show that in a stressful situation women have increased activity in brain regions that involve emotion. This increased activation is the result of stress and it lasts longer than in men, which means women remain nervous and worried for longer. This may explain why more women than men tend to have anxiety disorders and clinical depression.

Here are some tips for how you can take control and minimise stress in your life:

✔ **Declutter.** Everyone's busy. The trick is to balance your priorities. The first thing that you should look at is whether you really need to do everything that you're doing. Not everything you do is important; and you certainly don't need to do everything right now. When you take on too many things, you can find yourself constantly stressed or frazzled.

Make a decision to declutter your life. The first thing to do is to take an inventory. Evaluate how you spend your day. Next, think of everything that you don't need to do. Get rid of those activities. What do you have left on your list? Can you trim it down even further? Start by deciding on one item a day from your to-do list that you can eliminate, delegate, or ignore. Try to live each day by focusing on what's important rather than the multiple extra things that are unnecessary and leave you stressed out.

✔ **Take baby steps.** In the current digital age where information is so quickly accessible, you can easily expect that change should also be evident as fast. However, don't expect this to be the case. Make goals for yourself that you can easily achieve. Each week, list just one thing that you're going to change. Make your goal as concrete as possible. Instead of saying, 'This week I won't get stressed,' say, 'This week, I won't act in an aggressive manner and shout when I feel frustrated.' And make that happen.

✔ **Just say no.** If you're the type of person who finds it hard to say no to others, now's the time for change. Passive behaviour can lead to you ending up with extra work, feeling stressed out. and even resenting the person whom you can't turn down. Today's the time for change. If you find it too hard to say no outright, then you can say something like, 'Let me think about it.' You can also offer to do something that may not take up as much time but would still be helpful. Just remind yourself that only you can take care of your mental health – so if you find yourself over-committing to other people's requests, then it's time to say no.

✔ **Delegate.** Sometimes people say 'yes' to a responsibility, like being on a committee or hosting a party, when they're already stretched. If you find it hard to say no, try delegating the responsibility. Say 'I'm sorry that I can't host the party, but perhaps Mary is available to host it instead'. Who knows? You may even help someone uncover their hidden passions for doing an activity!

✔ **Stop multitasking.** Many reasons exist to stop multitasking. For starters, multitasking is an inefficient way to work because you have to constantly switch gears from one task to another. This constant switching can lead to stress. So first, make a list of priorities for each day. Then set aside time to complete one task at a time. For example, maybe you prefer to answer emails in the evening. So, if you can, close out your email during the day so you're not distracted.

✔ **Organise your time.** Set yourself time limits for tasks or activities so you don't end up spending more time on it than you should. If you're interrupted during a task and you're called away for something urgent, make a note of where you stopped and what remaining steps you have to accomplish. This makes it easier for you to come back, pick up where you left off, and finish what you need to do.

# Chapter 10

# Reaping the Rewards of Peace and Quiet

. . . . . . . . . . . . . . . . . . . . . . . . . . . . . . . . . . . . .

*In This Chapter*

▶ Creating a quiet space in your brain

▶ Making time to be quiet

▶ Finding out the benefits of meditation and prayer

. . . . . . . . . . . . . . . . . . . . . . . . . . . . . . . . . . . . .

*I*n the current digital age, thanks to Wi-Fi, BlackBerries and various other mobile devices, you never have to stop working! You can even check your email while you have a coffee at your local café. But do you really want the constant bombardment of noise and stress in your life?

Although the idea of a four-hour work week certainly isn't possible for most people, you can gain from turning off and stepping away from the daily grind in order to keep your brain functioning at its best.

## Using the Power of Silence

Silence doesn't always mean quiet. Though this may sound like a contradiction, silence in this chapter refers to much more than quiet. *Silence* refers to a sense of calm and rest for your brain (see Chapter 9 for the effects of stress and anxiety on the brain).

### Finding meaning in the noise

Noises surround you. Do you ever wonder how someone can follow a conversation in the roar of a party or a busy room? Well, scientists now have the answer. In order to understand more about how the brain processes sounds and determines what's meaningful from what's not important, scientists used *magnetoencephalography* (MEG) to measure brain activity during a series of different noises.

# The singing brain

Do you ever get the feeling that a tune is stuck in your head and you can't get it out? This sensation is known as *sound imagery* and can happen with everything from that broken record tune to someone's phone number. How does this information get stuck in the brain?

Researchers gave people two different types of songs to listen to – a familiar song and an unfamiliar song. Then the researchers took out chunks from the familiar songs and replaced them with silence. People didn't notice these silent gaps in the familiar songs although they did with the unfamiliar songs. The part of the brain associated with auditory processing (the *primary auditory cortex*) is highly activated when people hear songs that they know. The primary auditory cortex is located in the temporal lobe (see Chapter 2), which is in the left hemisphere of the brain.

When a song gets stuck in your head, you can't remember the words so sound imagery kicks in and just replays the parts that you know over and over again to fill in the gaps. If you want that tune to stop, the best thing to do is to look up the next line in the song and sing that as well!

So what helps a person makes sense of a conversation in a noisy place? You may be surprised to discover that understanding a conversation isn't all in the ears. The brain fills in the gaps of missing words to follow along a conversation. So even if you hear part of a word, your brain looks up possible matches and then, based on the context of the conversation, it fills in that word.

Scientists now know that the left hemisphere of the brain (which is also linked to language skills; see Chapter 2) helps people pick out meaningful sounds from random noises. When the brain is surrounded by noises from different sources, like on a busy street or in a noisy room, these signals compete with each other for attention. The brain uses a process called *simultaneous masking* to make sense of the noise and focus on what's relevant.

Studies have used MEG to test the involvement of the different parts of the brain. When scientists played a conversation to a person's left ear and background noises to the right ear, and then vice versa, in both cases, the left hemisphere showed the most brain activity. In other words, the left hemisphere works hard to focus on what's critical and masks the competing sounds and background noises.

## *Finding calm amidst the chaos*

Some people like to use a simple exercise to find an oasis of calm in their heads. You can try a modification of this exercise by following these steps:

1. **Turn off your phone, computer, and any other distractions that make a noise.**

2. **Sit down in a comfortable position.**

   You don't have to sit cross-legged on the floor. A soft chair or even the sofa is fine. If you don't feel too uncomfortable, try to sit with your back straight, though don't tense your shoulders.

3. **Close your eyes and focus on just one thought.**

   Don't try to analyse your thoughts and work through them. You may find it easier to focus on an object instead of your thoughts.

Just try this exercise for a few minutes at first until you feel comfortable. Then you can add on more time. The recommended time is a maximum of ten minutes.

## It's not just your ears; it's your brain

Elderly people commonly struggle with their hearing. But putting this difficulty all down to a loss of hearing is a misconception. The brain is also the culprit.

In one study researchers used magnetic resonance imaging (MRI) to scan the brains of young and old adults when they heard a series of words. To make things harder for the adults, the researchers gave them different words that were harder to understand.

The researchers then scanned the participants' brains and measured the volume in the parts of the brain related to understanding speech and attention. It comes as no surprise that the older adults had a harder time making sense of the warbled words compared to the younger adults. What's surprising is that even after the researchers took into account the possibility of hearing loss, the older adults were still struggling to hear.

Why? Because a part of the brain – the *auditory cortex* – had less volume. This part of the brain is responsible for processing sounds and was smaller in the older adults. This means that as people get older, a part of the brain linked to understanding sound gets smaller. Which may explain why even with the hearing aid turned up, Grandpa still has a hard time following the conversation.

If you find your mind wandering, reduce the time you spend in silence. The aim is to train your brain to focus on one thought (or one object) and filter out distractions. Starting with a manageable amount of time is important so you don't feel frustrated and abandon this activity.

## Making time for quiet

Health practitioners are now using meditation techniques with individuals who are experiencing early signs of Alzheimer's and dementia (read the section 'Overcoming the Daily Bustle with Meditation' in this chapter to find out more about how meditation and prayer benefit your brain).

But why wait until you start experiencing memory-loss difficulties? You can start meditating now by using these suggestions:

- ✔ **Don't wait.** Sometimes you find it easy to keep putting off spending a few moments alone in contemplation. But don't wait. Schedule in as little as 10 to 20 minutes each day to spend time on your own reflecting and mentally preparing for the day ahead. Just as your body needs food to survive, your brain experiences tremendous benefits from having those quiet moments each day.

- ✔ **Music helps.** Calming your brain down can be hard, especially if you're in the midst of a stressful situation. Some people find that music can be very helpful in putting aside thoughts related to stress. Think of a song that's meaningful to you. Find a quiet place away from everyone else and just spend some time in contemplation.

- ✔ **Just ignore.** When those nagging, stressful thoughts sneak into your mind during your moments of contemplation, make an active effort to block them out. Remind yourself that you have allocated this time just to relax and put aside such thoughts that are weighing you down. The goal is to block negative and distracting thoughts (see Chapter 9 for more information on managing stress and anxiety). Ultimately, you find that your attention and concentration levels increase as a result of ignoring distracting thoughts as you contemplate.

## Overcoming the Daily Bustle with Meditation

In the daily grind of activities and responsibilities, your brain needs a break too. And it's not just sleep that's important. Finding ways to mentally relax and meditate can have tremendous benefits for your brain power:

- ✔ **Better attention.** Studies have found that even people who are new to meditation can benefit from spending as little as 30 minutes a day meditating. After eight weeks, people who'd meditated for 30 minutes daily had greatly improved concentration and attention skills. They were better able to focus on the tasks they needed to accomplish and complete them more quickly and accurately. Even when many demands on their time existed, the people who meditated were still able to focus better. Good news for those who say they have too much to do and too little time!

- ✔ **Sharper brain.** If eight weeks is too much of a commitment for you to achieve a more restful brain, take heart. A study revealed that after just four days of using a meditation technique called *mindfulness* (a non-judgemental awareness of the present) for 20 minutes, people did better on cognitive tests compared to those who didn't practise any meditation. The participants in the study were able to remember more information and process information faster even under stressful conditions. This increased performance demonstrates how adaptable the brain is and that you don't need years of practice to achieve the benefits of a sharper brain.

- ✔ **More grey stuff.** Not only does meditation help your brain work better, but scientists have also found that it can physically change your brain. People who meditate regularly have an increased thickness in the part of the brain (the *frontal cortex*) associated with memory, concentration, and attention. This means that meditation may be able to reverse some of the effects of aging in the brain. Different types of meditation have different impacts on specific regions of the brain, but the take-home message is the same – meditation can protect your brain from the aging process and keep it sharp for longer.

## What happens in the brain during meditation?

Whether you're asleep or awake, the brain generates some level of electrical activity (see Chapter 14 for more on sleep). One study examined the brain's electrical activity during meditation using *EEG* (*electroencephalography*), which records neurons firing in the brain. The researchers found an increase of *theta* brain waves in the frontal and middle parts of the brain (see Chapter 2 for more information on the brain). *Theta waves* are associated with relaxing – your brain's downtime when it's not directly engaged in a mental activity. When someone meditates, the brain is in a state of deep relaxation and calm. Meditation also impacts your physical response and the body relaxes during this time. *Alpha waves* are also present during meditation. They signal the fact that the brain is relaxing or is at rest.

*Delta waves*, which are associated with sleep, aren't present during meditation. *Beta waves*, which signal active concentration – the type of brain waves that are present when you're working hard on something – also aren't present during meditation. Meditation produces very specific brain wave patterns that are associated with relaxing and calmness, which is different from those associated with sleep patterns.

*Mindfulness meditation* is a training programme thought to boost cognitive performance. It's like mental aerobics to train your brain to focus attention and improve concentration skills. Relaxation is key, and you focus on your breath. If a thought strays into your head during the meditation, you acknowledge the thought but let it go and continue focusing on your breath.

The goal of mindfulness meditation is to train the brain to ignore distraction and focus on what's important. In a world where you face a constant stream of information, this skill is certainly very useful.

## *Boosting your visual memory with meditation*

When you see a picture for the first time, it's unlikely to stay in your head for very long. Most people don't retain visual images for very long. In fact, an image typically lasts just a few seconds. So don't feel too badly if you can't remember someone's face after just meeting them briefly.

However, studies show that some types of meditation can boost your visual memory – at least temporarily. For example, Buddhist monks who are deep in their meditative practice have exceptional visual memory skills and can even remember highly complicated images for hours.

But research has found that if you want to increase your visual memory skills through meditation, only a special type of meditation works – the type of meditation that involves focusing on features of an object and mentally recreating all the features in as much vivid detail as possible. The type of meditation that avoids focusing on a single thought, object, or experience (see 'Finding calm amidst the chaos', earlier in the chapter) doesn't seem to improve visual memory skills.

In a series of experiments, researchers asked different meditation practitioners (those who focused on a single image in rich detail versus those who didn't), as well as non-meditators to take some visual memory tests. For example, in one test the participants had to mentally rotate a 3D picture. In another test they looked at a picture and had to remember it and identify it later.

After completing the visual memory tests, the practitioners were asked to meditate for 20 minutes. The non-meditators were given the option to rest. Then all the participants completed the visual memory tests for the second time.

The interesting finding was that the practitioners who meditated using a strong and highly vivid image showed a dramatic improvement on the visual memory tests compared to the other practitioners and the non-meditators. The practitioners who focused on a single image may have used the visual memory part of the brain during meditation, which in turn enhances this part of the brain even when they're not in a meditative state.

# Changing Your Brain with Prayer

A clear link exists between spirituality and your brain. Both the activity of the brain (such as in the study that I describe later in this section) and the physical changes of the brain (see the earlier section 'Overcoming the Daily Bustle with Meditation') demonstrate that prayer and meditation are powerful ways of keeping your brain alert and even counteracting the negative effects of aging on your brain's performance.

Researchers studied a group of monks and nuns while they were deep in prayer. They found that the *frontal lobe*, which is associated with attention and working memory (see Chapter 2), was working harder than average in the monks and nuns. This pattern demonstrates that when deep in prayer, these religious people are highly focused and attentive to their thoughts.

Here are some things that you can do to cultivate a sense of focus and thankfulness:

✔ **Say a prayer.** Science has shown that prayer can make a huge difference to your own physical and mental health. Those who pray or meditate regularly experience lower blood pressure, lower heart rates, decreased anxiety, and decreased depression.

Your prayer doesn't have to be long or even structured. The important thing is to spend a few moments praying. Even better, pray with a friend so you can also experience her support (see Chapter 11 for more on how socialising benefits your brain).

✔ **Keep believing.** Studies have found that people who are spiritual are more likely to report feeling happy and content with life. This sense of optimism (which some refer to as faith or hope) offers a tremendous boost to your brain and can serve as a buffer during difficult and stressful times.

✔ **Be thankful.** End each day listing three things that you're thankful for. Feeling discouraged by what *didn't* happen in a day is sometimes so easy that people forget to be grateful for what *did* happen. So before your head hits the pillow say a few things out aloud about why you were happy that day. Who knows, you may even end up smiling in your sleep!

*Neurotheology* is the use of brain imaging techniques to understand how the brain works during spiritual experiences. Spiritual experiences have the most impact on the brain when they move beyond the ritual (simply reciting a prayer or saying a chant) and are actually associated with beliefs or ideas.

# How God changes your brain

*How God Changes Your Brain* is the title of a book by a leading neuroscientist. Trained as a medical doctor, Andrew Newberg uses the ingenious technique of using brain imaging to find out what goes on up there during prayer and meditation. And the results are ground-breaking.

One of the key questions that Newberg asks is this. Is the brain of someone who's been engaged in religious and meditative practices different from someone who hasn't been involved in these practices? The short answer is yes!

Looking at the brains of nuns and monks reveals exciting evidence that their brains really are different – they function better and are better at focusing on information and filtering out distractions. But a slight problem exists, and it's a chicken and egg question – were the nuns and monks' brains better than others' to begin with or did their brains adapt as a result of their immersion in prayer and meditation?

With nuns and monks, researchers can't go back in time to look at their brains before they began their religious practices. But researchers can do something else. They've asked people who aren't engaged in this lifestyle to start a programme to see whether the brain changes after a few months of engaging in a specific practice of prayer or meditation. The pattern is the same: the brain changes in the person who begins prayer or meditation.

Newberg tells the story of a young Native American boy who was angry with his friend for stealing something that he treasured. In retaliation, the boy wanted to go and beat up his friend. However, he felt a conflict. On one hand, he was angry and wanted to take action against his so-called friend. But on the other hand, he also wanted to forgive his friend and be compassionate to him.

So the boy went to his wise grandfather to ask him why he felt conflicted by these two different responses. His grandfather responded by telling the boy that in each person's mind two wolves exist – one that's compassionate and wants to forgive and another that's angry and wants to exact revenge.

After thinking about this story for a time, the boy then asks his grandfather, 'If they're fighting each other, which one will win?' And the grandfather looks at the little boy and responds, 'It's the one that you feed.'

Newberg uses this story to illustrate how each person has the capacity for two sides. Based on brain imaging evidence of the benefits of prayer, it seems worthwhile to 'feed' your spirituality to strength the part of the brain that's compassionate and forgiving.

# Chapter 11

# Keeping Your Brain Sociable

- - - - - - - - - - - - - - - - - - - - - - - - - - - - - - - - - - - - - - - -

*In This Chapter*

▶ Discovering the benefits of friendships for your brain

▶ Staying away from isolating behaviour

▶ Going digital to improve your brain

- - - - - - - - - - - - - - - - - - - - - - - - - - - - - - - - - - - - - - - -

*S*ocialising is probably one of most fun ways to train your brain. After all, who doesn't like spending time with people they like! Friends can open up your world to new experiences, share the burden of a difficult situation, and make you feel on top of the world.

This chapter provides many reasons why friendships are so important for your brain. I also list tips on how to maximise your social relationships.

## Letting Go of Anger and Loneliness

Anger and loneliness both lead to stress, anxiety, and depression, which have negative consequences for how your brain works. Scientists have found that anger compromises the brain's ability to make rational decisions (see Chapter 2 for more on the prefrontal cortex). Anger can also increase stress hormones, which can ultimately lead to depression and to loneliness.

Being isolated has really harmful effects. In fact, scientific research has demonstrated that shutting yourself away from social interaction can be as bad as these things:

✔ Smoking 15 cigarettes a day

✔ Being an alcoholic

✔ Not exercising

✔ Obesity (twice as harmful)

Studies have found that lonely people are twice as likely to get dementia and Alzheimer's disease later in life compared to people who aren't lonely. And I'm not just talking about physical loneliness. Even *emotional isolation* – the feeling of being alone rather than actually being alone – is a risk factor for Alzheimer's disease. The take-home message is that people are social creatures. You need social interaction. So even if you feel tired or stressed out, call a friend. Reaching out can make a big difference to your mental health.

# Making Friends and Losing Enemies

Social relationships, such as a network of family and friends, have a range of benefits, from influencing your physical health to helping you cope better with stress (see Chapter 10) and finding a purpose in life (Chapter 9). When someone feels connected to other people, he has an aim in life and a sense of responsibility. This means that he's more likely to look after himself so he can continue to be there for those in his social network. Research has found that this positive effect of relationships is evident for all ages, and not just older adults. So don't take your relationships for granted – they're keeping you and your brain healthy.

Friendships help the brain work better. One reason is that friendships offer positive peer pressure. Seeing your friends' lifestyles can motivate you to make healthy changes that also improve your mental health. In addition, friendships give you a sense of purpose and meaning. In stressful and difficult times, friendships provide the emotional support that can help combat depression and help you overcome your problems.

Friendships also provide cognitive and memory challenges. Through regular discussions and conversations, which can range from the weather, to politics, to family relationships, to current events, friendships expand your horizons and encourage you to think in different ways.

If you're over 50, another reason to keep up your friendships exists. Studies have found that your social environment is an important predictor of cognitive skills, such as memory and attention. In a study that lasted six years, researchers tracked the social connectedness of almost 20,000 people aged over 50 years old. Those who were in a stable and long-term relationship and had regular contact with their children, parents, and neighbours experienced less memory loss five years later compared to those people who were more isolated. This finding means that social integration – your friendships – preserve your memory.

Follow these suggestions of different things that you can do with a friend:

✔ **Have a laugh.** A simple thing like laughing releases hormones that combat stress and boost the brain. If you don't have a funny friend, even watching a humorous video has the same effects. Even better, watch a video clip of your friends, maybe something you made together on holiday or at a celebration.

✔ **It's good to talk.** You haven't made any plans yet for the weekend. What should you do? Will you spend the afternoon

- Meeting up with a friend to discuss the latest movie you watched?

- Doing the daily crossword on your own?

- Watching some television?

Your answer determines how well you help your brain work. Psychologists found that simply meeting up with a friend to talk gives your brain the same benefits as doing a brain stimulating activity like the crossword puzzle. So the next time you have a free afternoon, turn off the TV and spend time talking with a friend instead.

✔ **Join a class.** Doing an activity with people is a great way to combine several ways to boost your brain – socialising and learning something new. Whether you choose a pottery class, an aerobics class, or even a class on wine tasting, go with a friend. Not only can you share the experience with someone, but also you can talk about what you're learning. You get the social benefits of going with a friend, as well as mental benefits because you can swap notes on what you learned. (Chapter 18 gives you suggestions on ten activities that help your brain.)

# Staying Happy and Fostering Friendships

People who have positive and healthy relationships are happier. And happy people live for longer. Studies have found that happiness protects against falling ill. On the other hand, people who are unhappy a lot experience more stress, which reduces their immune system, which in turn makes them get sick more often. It seems that friendships (or having coffee with a friend) really can keep the doctor away!

Happiness is infectious! Studies on thousands of people have found that when someone's happy, the good feeling spreads not only to his friends, but also his friends' friends, and their friends' friends' friends. And this wonderful feeling isn't just temporary. Your happiness can cause a chain reaction that affects other people that lasts for up to one year. Think of the world as a giant web with you in the middle. Your feeling of happiness spreads to your closest friends and family members, and they pass the happiness on to their friends, and they pass the happiness on to their friends, and so on. So go ahead and smile – you really could be making someone's day.

Even better, you're getting smarter while you're spending time with your friends. Socially active people really are smarter. Researchers studied almost 4,000 people from 24 to 96 years old. They asked the people questions about their social interactions, such as how often they talked on the phone with friends, neighbours, and relatives, and how often they went out together to events (dinner, classes, and so on).

The researchers found that people who were more socially engaged did much better on a test of their cognitive skills. Even after the researchers took into account differences in physical health and daily physical activity levels, people who were more social were smarter.

Social interaction boosts brain function because it involves many behaviours that require memory and attention. You use these same mental skills in many cognitive tasks throughout the day, from making a mental checklist of errands to preparing for a meeting. When you're socially active, you're working these brain 'muscles' and getting them ready to use when you have to solve a problem.

Here are some tips on how you can pick happiness instead of anger:

- ✔ **Choose to be happy.** Thinking that happiness is something that just happens is easy. Some people are luckier than others. In fact, that's not true. Happiness seldom drops at your feet. Happiness is something that you must (and can) choose. Psychologists say that *intention* is the first step in the road to happiness. You must make a conscious decision to choose attitudes and behaviours that lead to happiness rather than unhappiness. Make happiness your goal. Find reasons to be grateful and surround yourself with others who are also thankful for their circumstances.

- ✔ **Train yourself to forgive.** This may sound trite but an overwhelming body of research demonstrates the power of forgiveness. The healing effects extend not just for your physical health (forgiving reduces stress, anger, hypertension – the list goes on), but also for your mental health (it prevents loneliness, depression, and so on). The next time you feel that someone's offended you, don't nurse your feelings to create bitterness and resentment (see more on why to avoid rumination in Chapter 9). Remember that when you forgive, you're taking preventative steps for your mental health.

Instead, follow these steps:

1. **Think of why you're offended.**

2. **Try to see things from the other person's perspective.**

3. **Remember a time when you did something to offend someone (maybe it was unintentional).**

4. **Make a decision to forgive the person who's upset you.**

   Don't just do this in your head – write down that you forgive the person. If you don't want to write to the person, then write in your diary as a reminder of your decision. Keep looking at what you wrote every time you feel angry about the offence.

✔ **Do something you love.** People are happiest when they're involved in something that they enjoy doing. When your mind is fully engaged, your brain releases *endorphins* – feel-good hormones. In contrast, leisure activities such as watching TV are linked with the lowest levels of happiness. So whether you're scrapbooking (see Chapter 8), cooking a meal (Chapter 12), or going for a run (Chapter 14), find a passion – and a friend to share your activity with – and enjoy!

# You're never too old to make friends

Ivy Bean was 104 years old when she passed away. Ivy's passing may have gone unnoticed except for her family and close friends. Instead, Ivy's death was commented on by Gordon Brown, Stephen Fry, and a host of other British personalities. How did Ivy, a sweet woman who'd lived in a nursing home for the last 12 years of her life, capture the public interest?

Ivy was an Internet sensation. After hearing about an elderly French woman who had a Facebook profile, Ivy, at the age of 102 years decided to join as well. At the time of her passing, she had almost reached the maximum number (5,000) of friends a person can have on Facebook!

Ivy regularly reported on the events of her day, her favourite food, and what she'd watched on TV. Ivy is an inspiration that at any age you can make friends. Instead of feeling sorry for yourself, get out and start setting up social connections that won't only change your physical health, but boost your brain power as well.

One of the best 'cures' for unhappiness is having close and meaningful friendships with people who offer care and support. Studies have found that people over 70 who have the strongest network of friends live much longer. And you're never too old, too young, too busy, too . . . (fill in the blank) to make friends. If you need some inspiration to get going, read the nearby sidebar 'You're never too old to make friends'.

# Socialising Your Brain Digitally

In the current digital age more and more people are turning to digital means to stay connected. From social networking sites, to online gaming, to Internet-based phones, everyone seems more connected. But does digital technology offer the same benefits for the brain as face-to-face interactions? Read the section on 'Social networking sites are A-OK' to find out more.

The way that people interact online, whether it be in a multiplayer game or on a social networking site, provides a clue to how social relationships develop. Some researchers suggest that you can identify social interaction in an online gaming environment by six categories. Some categories are positive – friendship, communication, and trade; others are negative – hostility, aggression, and punishment. Online gamers are more likely to return the favours of positive actions compared to negative ones. For example, if Player A declares that Player B is his friend, Player B does the same. But if Player A declares that Player B is his enemy, player B won't always retaliate.

As with most things – too much of a good thing can be bad. This statement is also true of video game playing. Although benefits of video games exist (see the following section and Chapter 5 to see how video games can improve your spatial skills), moderation is the key. Overuse of video games means playing can start interfering with real life. For example, college students who played for 14 hours a week reported a drop in their grades and their health. It's not surprising to know that the students' social life was also affected, because they spent most of their free time in front of a computer screen. Family relationships can also deteriorate because you trade time with them for time with virtual relationships. So if you want to reap the social benefits of digital media without the negative consequences, follow the tips that I list in the section, 'Social networking sites are A-OK'.

# Multiplayer computer games count as socialising

Good news for those who like multiplayer online games – studies have found that these games promote sociability. The games work more like your local café where you meet up with virtual friends, rather than a prison where you're alone in your corner. Think of multiplayer online games as your hangout where you can meet up with friends and share some good moments, all without leaving your living room.

Multiplayer online games provide *social bridging,* which means that they provide a place for social interaction and relationships beyond the workplace and the home. These types of social relationships aren't so much for emotional support but allow the player to meet people from different walks of life. If you enjoy online gaming, research has found that multiplayer games offer more positive consequences – including making new friends – than single-player games.

Although multiplayer online gaming is far from isolated and passive, downsides exist, particularly for those who spend long periods of time in front of the screen in exchange for developing real-world social relationships. But instead of labelling multiplayer online gaming as *good* or *bad*, perhaps it's time to evaluate how you engage with this digital media – is your interaction healthy or unhealthy? Read more in the section, 'Social networking sites are A-OK'.

# Social networking sites are A-OK

If you're concerned about your son or daughter using social networking sites, you have reason to stop worrying. Studies have found that virtual relationships mirror real-life relationships. Young people who are well-adapted with positive friendships also seek out positive relationships in social networking sites. However, those who have behavioural problems and easily get depressed tend to use social networking sites in a negative and even aggressive manner (such as leaving hostile comments or using profanities).

So if you're a parent of a well-adjusted young person, don't worry. Your child's behaviour on social networking sites is much like it is with real-life social relationships.

The key for a parent is to stay involved in what his child's doing. Be supportive instead of intrusive and keep an open dialogue. That way, you're aware of your child's friends, what he's doing, and what he may be involved in, especially in his online pursuits.

# Does Facebook make you smarter?

Social networking is changing the face of friendship. Though social networking sites are relatively new, one of the most popular ones, Facebook, boasts of more than 300 million active users with an estimated 6 billion minutes spent on Facebook every day across the world.

Some social psychologists suggest that as a result of virtual connections, people are forming new *tribes* or social groups online based on a shared interest. These new friendships may not offer the same deep level of support that family and closer friends provide, but they're very similar to the acquaintances that people make at their local café or pub. A clear benefit of these virtual social connections compared to those that you make at your local hangout is that they represent people from different walks of life and can broaden your social horizon.

Yet social networking isn't without its critics. Some people suggest that technology makes you less intelligent, from the ever-increasing reliance on word processing to help improve grammar, Blackberries to remind people of appointments, speed-dial so you don't have to remember phone numbers, and a universe of information available at the click of a mouse.

So what you do give up when you rely on new technology? Are the likes of Facebook and YouTube reducing your ability to engage in everyday life? In fact, the opposite may be true: technology can dramatically improve your working memory.

Apart from the novelty of connecting with people whom you haven't seen since you were 5 years old (for better or for worse!), Facebook can also promote a sense of social connectedness. Those who are cut off from others often become isolated and may miss out on many benefits within education and employment. Studies on elderly populations found that those who spent more time meeting up with friends or talking on the phone, experience less memory loss than their peers who were more isolated.

Technology is advancing quickly and more and more students use social networking sites. But what impact does this have on education? Can virtual social connections boost working memory? I looked at these questions in a recent study. A group of 16-year-olds filled in a questionnaire about how long they spent using social networking sites such as Facebook. I also measured the young people's IQ, working memory, and academic attainment. I found that those who used Facebook for more than a year had better working memory scores, as well as higher spelling and vocabulary scores. In contrast, using a more passive form of digital media like YouTube didn't increase any of the young people's cognitive skills.

The sense of belonging and social connectedness that people feel when using social networking sites such as Facebook releases a feel-good hormone, which bolsters working memory. Good news for schools that are integrating social networking sites into their programmes.

Here are some tips on how to stay involved:

*TRY THIS*

✔ **Set a limit.** Everything in moderation; nothing in excess. This statement couldn't be more true for digital technology, particularly online gaming. Many social benefits exist for multiplayer online games, but slipping into excess is easy. So to avoid overuse of gaming, set a clear limit for how much time you'll play a day. Studies have found that people who play for two hours each day experience negative consequences to their health and their social relationships. So the next time you go online to play, try setting a timer for one hour and be strict with yourself about logging off after the timer goes off.

✔ **Make your online interactions positive.** If you're the type of person who seeks out positive and healthy relationships in real life, then the chances are you do the same with your online relationships as well. However, if you find yourself drawn to potentially negative social situations, use your online social connections to break the pattern. Stop before you write something hostile or mean and think of something positive instead. If someone sent you an email or a message, what would you like to read? Something friendly? Something positive? Remember that the next time you press the Enter key to send an online message.

✔ **Get involved.** Not all digital media gives you the same benefits. My research has demonstrated that engaging in more active online pursuits, like social networking, is linked to greater cognitive skills, like higher IQ and better working memory (see Chapter 5), compared to doing something passive online like watching digital video clips or surfing the Internet. Passive activities make you switch off and don't have any positive benefits for your brain. So the next time you go online, get your brain involved too (read the nearby sidebar 'Does Facebook make you smarter?' for the full story).

# Part IV

# Getting Physical: Looking at Brain-Friendly Diet and Lifestyle

The 5th Wave                                    By Rich Tennant

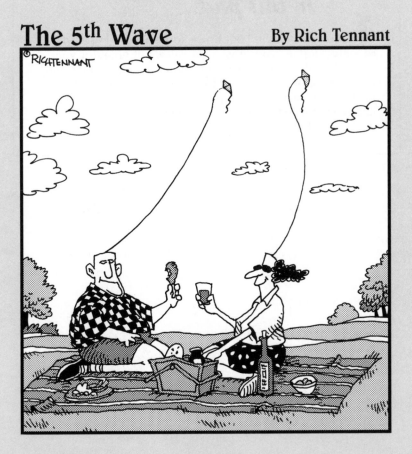

# In this part...

*I*n this part you find out how exercise and food aren't only good for your physical health, but great for your brain. You discover more about brain-boosting foods and what you should stay away from. Not all supplements and herbs increase your brain power. You see which have scientific evidence to improve your memory and which just drain your brain.

# Chapter 12

# Feeding Your Brain

## In This Chapter

▶ Getting nutrition for your baby

▶ Giving your child the best nutritional start

▶ Eating for your brain throughout your lifetime

*F*ood has a tremendous power over your brain, from reminding you of fun-filled childhood memories (Chapter 4) to relaxing frazzled nerves (Chapter 10). Yet most people probably view food as purely functional – something they have to do to keep their bodies moving. Eating is something you may do without too much thought, sometimes with friends at a swanky new restaurant; sometimes on your own in front of a TV. In this chapter, however, I highlight how food can actually change your brain from childhood to adult life.

Taking advice from a suitably qualified medical practitioner is always a good idea before making significant changes to your diet.

## Eating for Life: Nutrition in the Womb

Usually, during pregnancy a lifestyle change is the last thing on a woman's mind. The only change a pregnant woman wants to make is to put up her feet and enjoy the last few months of relative calm before the baby arrives. But picking the right foods offers great benefits for both you and your baby's brain. If making healthy choices means a change for you, do it – both you and your baby's brains will thank you.

### Craving Marmite

You've probably heard the stories of women who wake up their partners in the middle of the night and send them on a wild goose chase for some elusive food combination, such as chocolate-dipped pickles or Marmite on the special nut bread from that one shop they loved on holiday. The list goes on. Although most of the time these odd requests are just cravings, some cravings can be your brain's way of telling you that you're missing something from your daily food intake, such calcium or protein.

I'm not going to give you a list of essential nutrients that you need during pregnancy. Instead, what I'll do is tell you the top three brain boosters you can't (and shouldn't) live without during pregnancy. And I guarantee they're more important than Marmite!

✔ **Milk – it's not just for kids.** If you were never a milk drinker except for a few drops in your tea or coffee, then pregnancy is the time for change. Aside from the obvious benefits of calcium, which gives your baby stronger bones and teeth and better muscle and nerve functioning, milk provides other benefits too. Expectant mothers who drink milk during their pregnancy can lower the risk of multiple sclerosis (MS) in the child. You may be aware that symptoms of MS include tiredness, muscle weakness, and acute or chronic pain. But did you know that MS also affects your brain? MS sufferers also experience cognitive difficulties like depression (see Chapter 9 for more on changing your mindset) and problems in speech. Expectant mothers who drink less than one glass of milk a week are more likely to have children with a higher risk of MS. The benefits of milk come down to vitamin D. So next time you're thirsty, pass on the fizzy drinks and reach for milk instead (or vitamin D supplements – check with your doctor).

✔ **Iron isn't just for musclemen.** Iron is essential for brain development of the baby and serious cognitive consequences exist if the mother doesn't get enough iron. For example, iron deficiency in the growing baby in the womb results in learning and memory problems later in the baby's life. These negative consequences are often irreversible. So the take-home message is to give your baby the best start and make sure that you're getting enough iron.

Most pregnant women get folic acid and iron supplements from their doctor. But you can also get iron from food sources. Red meat is the best source, and the biggest source of iron from meat is an 8-ounce rump steak. If you're looking for a vegetarian source, you can get iron from grains and legumes – a mere quarter of a cup of bran flakes gives you the same amount of iron.

✔ **One, two, eat your omega 3.** Omega 3s are a type of poly-unsaturated fatty acids found in fish and different seeds. Although fat has a bad reputation, polyunsaturated fatty acids constitute one of four types of fats your body gets primarily through what you eat. And your baby needs it for her brain development. You may be familiar with common food sources of omega 3, such as oily fish (salmon and mackerel) and olive oil. But did you know that you can get omega 3 from spices that you probably have in kitchen? Some of these include cloves, basil, sage, oregano, and mustard seeds. Keep in mind that if your baby doesn't get enough omega 3 from what you're eating, she takes it from your own stores, which means that you can lose up to 3 per cent of your brain cells.

# Is pregnancy brain a myth?

So this week I've burnt the pasta (twice!), booked flights for the wrong day, put the milk away in the cupboard with the glasses, and locked the car and house keys in the car. If you asked me in my sixth month of pregnancy whether pregnancy brain is a myth, I'd say NO!

Some pregnant women blame such actions on the lack of sleep. However, it seems that I can't use sleep deprivation as an excuse for my forgetfulness. Studies have found that lack of sleep isn't actually linked to memory loss and forgetfulness in pregnant women.

Thankfully, a reason for my new (and unwanted!) absent-minded brain does exist. Scientific studies show that during pregnancy a woman's brain changes. For starters, the hippocampus, which is linked to spatial memory and long-term knowledge (see Chapter 7), actually shrinks during pregnancy. This means that a pregnant woman's sense of direction isn't always as reliable as it used to be.

Why does the pregnancy brain shrink? Brain shrinkage is the result of hormone changes during pregnancy, especially in the final trimester. Some hormone levels, such as progesterone and oestrogen, rise and fall during pregnancy. You need a perfect balance of these hormone levels to use working memory – your ability to incorporate new information with long-term knowledge stores. When oestrogens are very high, such as during the last trimester of pregnancy, working memory isn't as efficient. This makes simple tasks like remembering that the milk goes in the fridge (and not the cupboard) or juggling multiple tasks at work a little more difficult than usual.

Happily, brain size goes back to normal after the baby is born. Pregnant women can be confident of performing to their usual cognitive capabilities, but be aware that the pregnancy brain means that they may be more affected than usual when taking on additional responsibilities.

The message is a no-brainer, yet between 15 to 20 per cent of women smoke during their pregnancy. You've heard it before, but this message is so important that it bears repeating. Smoking during pregnancy results in serious risks for both you and your baby:

- Smoking mothers are likely to have babies who are premature and under-weight.

- Smoking also poses later consequences for children.

  - As the babies of mums who smoked during pregnancy grow up, serious consequences exist for the children's mental health.

  - Mothers who smoke during pregnancy put their children at greater risk of developing psychotic symptoms, such as hallucinations or delusions in their teenage years.

  - The exposure to tobacco in the womb can affect the brain by affecting impulsivity, attention, and even mental development.

## Resisting the sugary urge

If you're a food-lover then you may be tempted to think of pregnancy as a time to stock up on all your favourite foods, regardless of their calories or fat content. But before you throw caution to the wind, keep in mind the consequences for both you and your baby.

- **Like food?** Pregnant mothers who eat high-fat and sugary foods end up negatively affecting their baby's brain development. The babies' brain pleasure centres became progressively less responsive. This means they have a hard time saying no. As a result, these children can develop compulsive overeating habits and become vulnerable to obesity, and may display addictive-like behaviours in adulthood. Babies born to mothers on a high-fat diet during pregnancy have a greater weakness for sugary food compared to pregnant mothers on a standard diet.

- **Sugar high.** Gestational diabetes occurs in up to 10 per cent of pregnancies and is characterised by women who have high blood sugar during pregnancy. When a mother's blood glucose (sugar) is high during pregnancy, their child is more likely to have low insulin sensitivity, which is a risk factor for type 2 diabetes.

Researchers have uncovered evidence to show that piling on too many pounds in pregnancy may lead to future heart risks in the child. Although researchers are debating the ideal weight gain in pregnancy, most agree that it should reflect how much the baby is growing, as well as a healthy weight for the mother.

# *Eating for Life: Nutrition in Childhood*

The good news is that you can give your child a head start in life by giving her a healthy and nutritious home environment.

Many passing fads claim to have the magic combination of nutritional value that your child needs for success. Unless the supplement you're taking is approved by an official agency (like the Food Standards Agency in the UK or the Food and Drug Administration in the US), avoid it. Many supplements on the market masquerade as 'vitamins' and don't have approval from government bodies. Don't be taken in by the advertising on these supplements – you could end up doing more harm than good. The following advice is based on scientific research, rather than current food fads.

## *Fishing for your brain*

If you needed convincing on the merits of serving fish to your child, this study may change your mind. When scientists looked at teenagers who ate fish more than once a week, they found that these students had a much higher IQ score than their peers who ate fish only once a week (see Chapters 6 and 7 for more on IQ tests).

How do omega-3 fatty acids help your child's brain? Docosahexaenoic acid (DHA) and eicosapentaenoic acid (EPA) are polyunsaturated fatty acids of the omega-3 family. Your body can't make these essential nutrients, so you must obtain them from the food you eat. DHA is a major building block of the brain, as well as the nervous system. A lack of omega-3 fatty acids leads to a range of cognitive problems in childhood, including learning difficulties, poor memory, and lack of concentration.

Scientists are debating whether fish oil supplements can provide the same benefits. Some studies show that children who receive fish oils in supplement form show more brain activity in areas linked to attention compared to those who receive a placebo.

Be careful of the supplement and only buy from a trusted source. If you'd rather not use supplements, then give your child one serving of oily fish a week to see benefits.

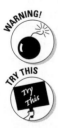

So here are some fishy delights that are best for your child:

   ✔ **Salmon.** Salmon tops the list of the best fish for your brain. But it's not just any salmon that does the trick. Wild salmon is much better than farm-raised salmon. Not only is wild salmon an excellent source of omega 3, but it also has a low amount of mercury. Fish caught in the wild have a chance to grow and develop, which means that their muscles and tissues are stronger. This means that you're getting a better fish.

✔ **Sardines.** This is another fish that's an excellent source of omega-3 fatty acids. Like salmon, sardines have extremely low levels of mercury. However, keep in mind that sardines canned in oil can be high in cholesterol.

✔ **Tuna.** You can gain many health benefits from eating tuna, including canned tuna. For example, tuna is an excellent source of omega-3 fatty acids and has been linked with lowering the risk of Alzheimer's.

Although I include tuna in this section, a caution comes with this point. Canned tuna can be dangerous for pregnant women due to the high levels of mercury found in it (see the earlier section 'Eating for Life: Nutrition in the Womb' for more on dietary advice during pregnancy to boost your baby's brain power). Mercury is a toxin that can damage the baby's brain during gestation and some doctors suggest that pregnant women avoid tuna altogether.

If you have a child who's a picky eater, fish can be a difficult option to serve. However, you can make fish more appetising (even if you child isn't convinced of its brain value). I provide some tips in the section 'Dealing with picky eaters'.

The best thing is to introduce fish when children are young because then it's much easier to encourage healthy eating habits that last a lifetime.

## Dealing with picky eaters

Children can be notoriously difficult to please, especially when it comes to food. My 3-year-old is no exception. So, whenever I'm introducing a new food, I follow three rules:

✔ **Incorporate the food with an exciting story.** My little boy loves stories about pirates and dinosaurs, so when I made fish cakes with salmon for the first time, we told a great pirate adventure story as we were eating. It worked really well and now he has positive associations with eating salmon because he enjoyed the story so much.

If you don't like making up stories then pop to your nearest library and get books that your child will enjoy reading or that you can use to link the new food with the story. For example, one mother talked about reading the classic *Green Eggs and Ham* by Dr Seuss when she introduced spinach and eggs to her children. They loved it! But it doesn't have to be books – the key is distraction. Provide children with another activity that they enjoy doing when you introduce a new food. If your child likes colouring then get her a new colouring book to do when you present her with a meal of sardines. This way, whenever your child thinks of the new food, that thought is positive because she pairs it with an activity she enjoys.

✔ **Be a model.** If your child sees you enjoying fish then she's more likely to eat it as well. Serve the new food during a meal that you eat together as a family. When your child sees everyone else enjoying the food too she'll feel more interested in trying it. Make a big deal about how much you're enjoying the food.

✔ **Wait until your child's hungry.** Avoid giving children a snack or a drink (water is fine) too close to mealtimes. This way a child is more likely to look forward to each mealtime and try new foods.

It also helps to pair up a new food with an old favourite. If your child loves tomatoes, serve her sardines with a lovely home-made tomato sauce. Or why not try an old favourite like fish and chips with salmon instead?

Don't try to introduce more than one new food at a time. This can overwhelm your child and she's likely to push it away.

## Snacking right for a better brain

Researchers have suggested that diet in childhood is the culprit for behaviour problems. There's been a lot of research in this area, but the key to remember is that the wrong food does *not* cause attention-deficit hyperactivity disorder (ADHD), although it can certainly worsen negative behaviour. If you're a parent and are concerned about your child's behaviour at home and at school, this section provides advice on how to manage behaviour through diet.

✔ **Don't add additives.** Additives are food colourings and preservatives that are often found in highly processed and sugary foods. If you read the label on foods you may see items like FD&C Yellow (E numbers). Clear evidence shows that food additives aggravate hyperactive and impulsive behaviours in young children (3-year-olds) up until middle childhood (10-year-olds), even in children without a diagnosis of ADHD. Increased hyperactivity leads to learning difficulties, especially in relation to reading, which can jeopardise your child's success in school.

✔ **Skip the sweets.** On average children consume about 2 pounds of sugar per week. Take a look at the size of your sugar packet the next time you go grocery shopping. That's a huge amount of sugar and much more than your child needs. Too much sugar can lead to hyperactivity and impulsivity. When you think of these behaviours, images of children bouncing off the walls may come to mind. But it can be much worse. A high sugar intake can also lead to destructive and aggressive acts, such as throwing or kicking things, and even damaging property. Younger children are most affected by the dreaded 'sugar high'. So although having a treat every so often is nice, keep sugary foods as just that – a treat, not a regular fixture of your child's diet.

✔ **Eating the good fat.** Earlier in this chapter I talk about fatty acids (in 'Fishing for your brain'). Omega 3 is also great for your child. However, your body can't produce these types of fatty acids, which means that you must get them from food. Studies have found that children with low levels of omega 3 are more likely to display behaviour problems, such as hyperactivity. Other side effects of a shortage of fatty acids include increased risk of eczema, allergies, and asthma – all of which you can alleviate by increasing your child's intake of fatty acids. The section 'Fishing for your brain' in this chapter provides tips on how to include fatty acids in your child's diet.

Knowledge is power. Studies have found that groups of parents who have less information on ADHD and how diet affects their children are less likely to seek support and treatment. Don't wait until it's too late to give your child the support she may need. As a parent you can provide the best start by ensuring that your child's diet is healthy and nutritious, rather than loaded up with processed and sugary foods.

Fructose and glucose are both forms of sugar that your body needs. They're forms of carbohydrates that your body converts into energy. Your body doesn't just use this energy for physical activities, but also for mental tasks. When sugar levels are low, decision-making skills and reasoning abilities can be affected. So if you should avoid sugar from processed food, like chocolate bars and sweets, where should you get your sugar? Well, fructose and glucose are different. Fructose is found in fruits, fruit juices, and some vegetables like tomatoes. On the other hand, glucose is found in most carbohydrates (this includes rice, pasta, and potatoes). It's best to eat glucose-rich foods at the start of the day when your body can convert them into energy for your body and your brain. If you eat glucose-rich foods at the end of the day, your body stores them as fat instead of converting them into energy.

## Breakfast first

If mornings are rushed at your house and you barely have time to eat anything, think about changing your routine. Numerous scientific studies demonstrate that breakfast really is the most important meal for your brain. One such study showed that students who didn't eat breakfast or just had a drink struggled on tests of memory and attention. Their performance grew even worse by mid-morning. In contrast, even having cereal helped the students to focus throughout the morning. Another study showed that students who eat breakfast regularly have higher test scores than their classmates who skip breakfast.

If you do have time to prepare breakfast for your child before school, consider foods that won't only give your child the energy she needs until lunchtime, but that also powers her brain. If possible, save the sugary breakfasts, like muffins and pancakes, for the weekend. Oats and bran cereals are a great energy source for the brain, and you can make them more exciting by adding yogurt or your child's favourite fruit as a topping. If your child needs something sweet, avoid sugar and try honey instead. Eggs are another great breakfast food for your child. If your child needs inspiration, trying reading the Dr Seuss classic *Green Eggs and Ham* the night before. Another trick that I use with my little one is to make an omelette into different shapes and tell a story. Usually, he's so engaged in the story that he doesn't have time to complain about the eggs!

# Developing Eating Habits for a Lifetime

Most of you have probably been on a diet at some point in your life. Whether it was for an event you wanted to look good for or health reasons, most people can relate to the trials and tribulations of calorie counting. Yet calorie counting and bouncing from one diet plan to another isn't really a good way to live life. You probably know that having a food plan that's part of your lifestyle is much more effective. In this section I list foods that research shows are an essential part of any lifestyle. Don't worry; you don't have to eat like a rabbit to keep your brain at its best!

## Juicing for life

Juice bars have recently sprung up all over, and nowadays it's not hard to find one, even at a small airport. What's so great about juices? And how can they benefit your brain? For starters, juices are packed with vitamins, which have a host of benefits for your body and your brain.

Juices also give you your 'five a day' in a quick and easy method. Many people have an odd assortment of fruits and vegetables lying around the kitchen, and juicing lets you throw these all together. You can experiment with all sorts of combinations: celery and apple, cabbage and mango, broccoli and raspberry – the list is endless. You don't even need any cooking skills!

Here's a list of some fruits that should be at the top of any juicing list:

- **Pomegranates.** Recently, pomegranate juice has become very popular. Pomegranate juice is very pleasant to drink and studies confirm that unlike most food fads this one really does live up to its hype. For starters, pomegranates are a 'superfood', which means that they're rich in antioxidants, more so than other fruit. Pomegranate juice is great from pregnancy to adulthood. At one end of the lifespan, expectant mothers who drink this juice can help the baby's brain to resist brain injuries resulting from low oxygen supply. At the other end of the lifespan, studies confirm that pomegranate juice can prevent Alzheimer's disease, helping people stay sharp in old age.

- **Prunes.** If pomegranates are the 'trendy' fruit, people often think of prunes as distinctly unfashionable. Most people associate prunes with alleviating constipation and other related bladder conditions. But did you know that prunes are also good for your brain? Prunes contain vitamin A, which not only boosts your body's defence system but also helps brain cells repair themselves quickly.

  You can make your own prune juice by soaking 1 cup of prunes in 5 cups of water for four hours. Remove any seeds, puree, and enjoy.

- **Be 'grapeful'.** Grape juice contains high levels of flavonoids, which work to lower blood pressure and increase levels of good cholesterol. Studies have found that grape juice can improve memory and coordination. If you're already a fan of grape juice, make sure that you're drinking juice made from red or purple grapes because these are packed with brain-boosting goodness. One study even found that grape juice was better for your heart than cranberry or orange juice.

- **Colour me blue.** Blueberries are another superfood and are rich in vitamin C and potassium (which helps bones). Clinical trials found that 2 cups a day is enough to boost learning and brain power. Even frozen blueberries deliver the same benefits to your brain, so you can enjoy them all year long.

## The eggy truth

What's the story on eggs? One minute you're told that they're great for you, the next minute you hear that you should avoid eggs. And now it seems that more is better.

Researchers previously thought that eating eggs raised cholesterol levels. However, studies now confirm that for average individuals, eating up to two eggs a day poses no health risk at all.

The benefits of eggs are plain to see – they're rich in vitamins (vitamins A, B, D, and E), most of which are from the egg yolk. They're also rich in omega-3 fatty acids, which I talk about throughout this chapter. Pregnant women also benefit from eggs because they help the baby's brain development.

So what are you waiting for? Get scrambling, poaching, boiling, or frying. Whatever suits your taste!

 Be aware of the sugar content in ready-made juices. Some juices add so much sugar that a single glass can exceed the daily recommended dose. Read the contents to make sure that no sugar is added. Also try to avoid juices with sweeteners or aspartame, because these have been found to be bad for your health. If possible, make your own juice at home. This way you can be creative with your chosen combinations of fruits and vegetables and know that you're not adding extra sugar. Why not add a vegetable you don't eat often (maybe kale or spinach) with a favourite fruit. If you find fresh juice hard to stomach without sugar, add a little honey.

## *Making meat count*

You may have heard of the Atkins diet, which requires the person to cut out all sugar (including fruit) but allows lots of protein and fat, including steak and bacon. Although I'm not advocating the Atkins diet (or any other diet!), a protein-rich diet has merits.

 Eating protein encourages your brain to produce different chemicals to keep you energised and stay alert. But you don't need too much of it. Protein-rich foods should only make up 10 to 15 per cent of your daily calories. Chicken and lean meat provide the best sources. Vegetarians can get their protein fix from dairy products, legumes, and nuts.

 As with most good things, you pay a price with a protein-rich diet. Red meat can be high in cholesterol, which affects your health and your brain. Scientific studies have found that people on a diet that's high in saturated fat and cholesterol are more likely to experience memory loss. In particular, their working memories – the ability to remember and manipulate information – are very poor. How does such a diet affect your brain? This type of poor diet results in an inflammation in the brain. This inflammation affects memory skills, as well as physical functioning such as vision and hearing. The key is to use moderation and limit red meat to once a week.

## Brain foods in your cupboard

If you still have the view that eating healthy is like taking medicine, here are some brain foods that'll definitely put a smile on your face.

- **Black gold.** Tea drinkers, it may be time for a change. It's coffee's turn to shine. This simple and ubiquitous drink is incredibly rich in vitamins, minerals, and antioxidants – all of which give your brain a boost. In fact, coffee is such a great brain food that studies have shown that people who drink it regularly may actually reduce the risk of mental decline and Alzheimer's and dementia. Choose freshly ground coffee to get these benefits, rather than powdered coffee. If you can, swapping your cappuccino for an espresso is the best way to get your brain food – espresso is pure and full of brain-boosting properties. But do use moderation – too much caffeine has its negative effects (see Chapter 13).

- **Sweet tooth.** Chocolate is another food that you can smile about. The cacao bean – what chocolate is made from – has been hailed as a fantastic brain food. The cacao bean in its pure form is best. Dark chocolate with a high percentage of cacao solids is the next best thing. Milk chocolate contains too much sugar and too little cacao solids, and white chocolate contains no cacao solids at all. So before you indulge, make sure that you select chocolate that has at least 70 per cent cacao content. Otherwise all you're getting is the sugar, fat, and artificial flavourings, with none of the benefits.

- **Nutty delights.** Walnuts are touted as brain food because they're packed with omega-3 fatty acids. A mere quarter of a cup of walnuts provides over 90 per cent of the recommended daily intake of omega-3 fatty acids. Almonds and pistachios are another example of a brain nut. So get cracking and sprinkle these nuts over your oats, yogurt, and salads.

# Chapter 13

# Looking at Stimulants: Drugs and Caffeine

*I*n this chapter I discuss different types of stimulants. Most people are aware of the benefits of caffeine and the pitfalls of alcohol. Yet what's the trade-off – what potential harmful side effects are you subjecting your brain to for your daily cup of Java? And is it worth taking stimulants? This chapter looks at these questions and more.

## Pepping Up Your Brain

The most common method that people use to pep up their brain is to drink coffee. Coffee's caffeine content acts as a *stimulant*, which means that it speeds up your brain's activities to help you focus. But these effects never seem to last for very long, and by your second or third cup you may find yourself jumpy, anxious or even irritable. So what's the balance in harnessing the benefits of caffeine without the drawbacks? In this section I look at this issue in more detail.

### Keeping your brain sharp: What works and what doesn't

Caffeine is like a double-edged sword. On the one hand, caffeine has some positive effects on your brain. For example, some studies show that caffeine causes increased brain activity in the frontal lobe, which is linked to working memory (see Chapter 2 for more information on how the brain works). People who've had a small amount of caffeine perform better on memory tasks.

But on the other hand, caffeine has drawbacks. For example, long-term use of caffeine can be counter-productive and impair long-term assimilation of information. In particular, long-term caffeine consumption can affect the hippocampus and how it works to integrate new information. It can also increase the frequency of 'tip-of-the-tongue phenomenon' (see Chapter 6 for more on this topic). So although caffeine can help some aspects of your memory, it can also impair other aspects of cognitive skills, such as the acquisition of new information.

Caffeine tolerance can develop very quickly. All you need is to drink 400 milligrams of coffee three times a day for seven days. Although caffeine can perk you up, it can leave you feeling even more fatigued and drowsy. Your body experiences a drop in serotonin, which can cause anxiety, make it difficult to concentrate and resulting in the loss of motivation. Some people refer to these feelings as the *caffeine crash*. Not only does your brain experience a crash, but your body also experiences withdrawal symptoms like headaches and pains in the joints. Usually, having a cup of coffee is enough to banish these unpleasant effects.

Here are some ways in which you can enjoy your caffeine in moderation.

✔ **Make mine a single.** If you love your coffee, you may want to think about limiting it to one cup instead of two. Studies have found that cognitive skills improve after just one cup (8 ounces) of coffee. However, those who drank two cups ended up more irritable with a faster heart rate. So use moderation and ditch those extra cups of coffee – you don't need them and they certainly won't make your brain work better.

✔ **Tea for me.** Tea, green tea in particular, is one way to get your caffeine boost without all the negative side effects of addiction and withdrawal. Read the section 'Taking a cup of green tea a day to keep the doctor away' in this chapter to find out more.

✔ **Read the label.** If you're trying to cut down on your coffee intake, be aware that caffeine is found in a lot of other drinks and products. Of course, you probably know that tea and energy drinks contain varying amounts of caffeine. But most fizzy cola drinks have caffeine, too. If you have a cold, check the box – some medicines also have caffeine in them. Chocolate lovers may know that caffeine is present in chocolate, so eat it in moderation and not before bed if you don't want to stay awake!

Caffeine can have negative effects during pregnancy. Women who drink two or more cups of coffee are twice as likely to miscarry their babies compared to women who don't consume any caffeine during the pregnancy. It's not just the caffeine in coffee that increases the risk of miscarriage – caffeinated drinks (five 12-ounce or 350-millilitre cans of caffeinated drinks per day), such as fizzy drinks, tea, and even hot chocolate, can result in the same risks. As little as two cups of coffee a day can also affect the baby's heart development and result in poorer heart function throughout the child's life. So if you're pregnant and you can avoid caffeine, do it.

## Avoiding the caffeine dip

Caffeine's effect on the brain is almost immediate – in as little as ten minutes you can start to notice an increased level of alertness in your brain functioning. This effect usually lasts up to three hours, but in some cases the effect can remain for up to five hours, depending on your age and metabolic rate.

So how do you avoid the dreaded caffeine dip? Here are some tips on what to watch out for:

- ✔ **Beware the caffeine smiles.** Your caffeine shot does more than just taste good. It also increases your dopamine levels in your brain (your pleasure centre). So you keep drinking coffee because the caffeine in it activates your brain's pleasure centre, and the caffeine can be addictive. But when the buzz wears off you start feeling tired and down, and, of course, crave more coffee.

- ✔ **The caffeine sleep.** The purpose of your caffeine shot is to make your brain more alert. But be aware that if you drink too much caffeine near bedtime, you can, of course, stay awake. Some people, however, are still able to sleep even after drinking large amounts of coffee. However, they're not able to reach deep sleep (see Chapter 14 for more on the effect of sleep on your brain). Despite getting eight hours of sleep, they're still tired the next day and are more likely to be irritable, which, of course, impacts how well their brain can work.

- ✔ **All an illusion?** In a large study researchers gave one group of people caffeine and gave another group a *placebo* (a substitute that looked like coffee, but didn't contain any caffeine). The researchers found that the two groups performed at the same level when they were tested on tasks that measured how alert they were. People who report the caffeine high are actually just experiencing the coffee reducing their withdrawal symptoms and not actually an increased level of alertness.

✔ **The caffeine-filled decaf.** It's hard to remove the caffeine content completely from a coffee bean. Someone who drinks five cups of decaffeinated coffee gets the same levels of caffeine from one cup of caffeinated coffee. So if you have to cut out caffeine because of hypertension or an anxiety problem, you may want to stay away from your usual decaf coffee.

Frequent coffee drinkers need caffeine to bring their mind back to balance. When they don't have coffee, they start to experience withdrawal symptoms, including tiredness and anxiety. When frequent coffee drinkers get their coffee shot, the caffeine just reverses these effects rather than actually increasing their brain's alertness. In other words, the alert feeling that some get after coffee is just the caffeine bringing them back to their normal level of alertness.

# Relaxing Your Brain

Sometimes the brain needs to wind down and relax. In this section I discuss how you can keep your brain alert without the caffeine highs and lows.

## Taking a cup of green tea a day to keep the doctor away

If you were considering a move away from caffeine for the sake of your brain then green tea is the way forward. Green tea can boost your brain power without the caffeine withdrawal jitters.

In a study of people aged 70 and over, those who drank green tea had higher scores on tests of memory, spatial orientation, and direction, compared to coffee or black-tea drinkers. All it took was as little as two cups of green tea a day for better cognitive skills. When the researchers compared the performance of those who drank green tea daily with those who drank it three times a week, the daily drinkers had double the brain power – their scores were twice as high. However, if you can't stomach that much green tea in one day, don't despair. Even drinking green tea a few times a week is better than not at all.

What's so great about those leaves? Well, two things in particular. First, green tea contains *polyphenols* – a chemical that's a powerful antioxidant responsible for lifting up your mood, as well as acting as a buffer against Parkinson's disease (which impairs motor skills and speech). The polyphenols also boost the availability of dopamine, which is crucial for mood enhancement and is involved in helping muscles move smoothly. When someone suffers from Parkinson's, their dopamine production isn't functioning as it should, which results in muscle tremors. Polyphenols can increase dopamine levels and protect individuals against the negative effects of dopamine 'malfunction'.

Another fantastic ingredient in green tea is *tannin*, which has been found to have similarly wonderful brain-boosting ingredients. In particular, tannin can prevent brain damage that invariably occurs after a stroke. The tannin found in green tea helps the body repair itself to keep the brain working after head trauma. Of course, I'm not suggesting that drinking copious amounts of green tea is enough to rebuild the brain, but it can play an important role.

## Calming your brain

Stress and anxiety can affect the way the brain works (read more about how to calm your brain in Chapter 10). Although most people do feel anxious about certain things, feeling anxious all the time (chronic anxiety) isn't the norm. If you're experiencing symptoms such as frequent headaches, sweating, or hypertension that manifest in high-pressure situations, see your doctor right away.

Follow these tips to keep your brain calm and healthy:

✔ **Avoid sugary and processed foods.** In Chapter 12 I discuss how sugar is not brain food. Sugar can also affect your mental health. If you can't completely cut out processed foods, which contain a lot of sugar, try to limit them as a treat on the weekends, instead of making sugary foods part of your daily allowance. Examples of sugary and processed foods are muffins and chocolate bars. But most foods, including some labelled as 'health food', can contain more sugar than your body needs. So just check the label to make sure that your body is getting the right fuel for your brain. Recommended daily amounts are usually listed in a separate column to the actual contents of the food on labels, so compare the two to make sure that your intake doesn't exceed this amount.

✔ **Boost your grains.** Some people prefer to avoid medication and rely on a natural way to calm the brain. A food plan rich in complex carbohydrates can achieve that. Pick foods that are rich in whole grains, such as lentils and bran.

✔ **Drink your juice.** Drink citrus juices in particular – like orange juice. But try to get fresh juice and not processed or sweetened juice. Add a squeeze of orange to your salad; throw in some orange wedges into your salad or even your chicken dish; or, at the very least, add some to your water. Read Chapter 12 for more ideas on how juice can help your brain.

## Anxiety and the brain

Chronic anxiety is linked with a drop in *gamma-aminobutyric acid* (GABA) – a 'relaxing' chemical. GABA works to calm (instead of excite) electrical impulses in the brain. Scientist can measure electrical activity in the brain, and they've found that two waves in particular link to anxiety:

✔ *Beta waves* are the fastest of the four brain waves and are generated when the brain is mentally engaged in an activity. This can be when you're learning a new language, working on a presentation, or even arguing your point with a friend.

✔ *Alpha waves* represent the opposite activity of beta waves – they indicate when the brain is at rest. This may be during a time of reflection or meditation (see Chapter 10 for more on this topic).

Scientists suggest that GABA lowers beta waves, which can lead to 'racing thoughts'; and raises alpha waves, which contribute to feelings of calm and relaxation.

A natural supplement considered 'generally safe' by the Food and Drug Administration (FDA) in the US is *theanine*. This naturally occurring amino acid is found in green tea and has a calming effect without bringing about drowsiness. Scientific studies found that theanine increases alpha waves in the brain, which are indicative of serene and peaceful moments.

Although you can find theanine supplements in health food stores, use caution in the actual supplement you choose and the amount you take. Only buy supplements that have Food and Drug Administration or Food Standards Agency approval and be aware of claims on drinks that include theanine to relax you. Nutritionists say that a reasonable daily amount of is 20 milligrams a day (roughly two cups of green tea, depending on the strength of the leaves). However, some supplements contain up to 50 milligrams and even recommend taking 100 milligrams of theanine daily. Taking large doses like this can impair your judgement and induce the same tranquilising effect as alcohol – not a good idea if you're driving or engaging in any activities that require your full attention!

# Medicating Your Brain

Popping a pill seems so much easier than actually doing something to keep the brain active. But before you reach for the medicine cabinet, be aware that no conclusive evidence proves the benefits of 'smart drugs'. Some studies show a boost in memory skills and performance on cognitive tests, but others show no effects at all.

In this section I list a few most commonly available (and legal!) drugs for your brain.

## *Popping pills: Can they keep your brain sharp?*

Do brain pills exist? And if such a thing as brain pills exists, do they work?

The term *nootropics* refers to *smart drugs* – drugs thought to enhance memory, attention, motivation, and even intelligence. Smart drugs work by increasing oxygen supply to the brain and stimulating different neurochemicals for efficient cognitive functioning. However, an important qualifier exists – the long-term effects of nootropics haven't yet been determined. In other words, although smart drugs may improve your cognitive skills in the short term, no one quite knows the possible damage they may do to the brain in the long term.

Here are some examples of prescription medications that increase attention.

✔ **Stimulants.** As the name suggests, stimulants work to 'up' your brain power. These drugs function to increase alertness, keep you awake and generally increase arousal states in the brain. In this chapter I've already talked about the effects of caffeine in the form of coffee and energy drinks. Some medications do include caffeine in the list of ingredients and caffeine tablets are also available.

✔ **Modafinil.** This drug is only available with a legal prescription in the UK. Modafinil is most often used to treat sleep disorders. More recently, it's also been found to be effective in treating Parkinson's disease and ADHD. Modafinil works to combat the need for sleep and delay the resultant effects of tiredness. However, the long-term effects of this drug aren't known and side effects include irritability, anxiety, nervousness, and insomnia, and the drug may even result in fatalities.

✔ **Methylphenidate.** Doctors commonly prescribe methylphenidate to individuals with a diagnosis of ADHD. You can only get methylphenidate on prescription and the dosage varies depending on the individual and the symptoms. The drug works to help the individual focus more clearly. It's not recommended for those under 6 years of age and the benefits of methylphenidates disappear after the individual stops taking it. In other words, methylphenidates are almost always a lifetime commitment. Although doctors prescribe methylphenidates widely, research is ongoing regarding the long-term effects and potential for abuse.

# Methylphenidate for all?

Drug companies aren't allowed to market their products off-label; this means that you can't use the drug for a purpose other than for what it was intended. Yet a growing number of people are using medication like methylphenidate to boost their energy levels and help them focus for longer periods of time. Surveys of college students found that as many as 25 per cent of students use methylphenidates to give them a competitive edge in their academic pursuits.

With a prescription, the dosage is moderated and adjusted for each individual. However, in cases of methylphenidate abuse, people take a higher amount than they should or even take it without a proper prescription. Although it may seem like an easy shortcut, the consequences of methylphenidate abuse far outweigh the short-term benefits. For starters, methylphenidate is highly addictive – just as much as amphetamines and methamphetamines (which are both classed as illegal drugs). The addictive nature of methylphenidate can result in dangerous long-term consequences. Feelings of paranoia, an irregular heartbeat, and increased likelihood of heart failure and seizures are all conditions you can look forward to with an addiction to methylphenidate.

As with all medication, seek your doctor's advice. Never take more than the recommended dosage and only use the medicine for its recommended purpose.

## *Staying away from brain drainers*

If you'd rather stay away from pills then natural herbal supplements may offer similar benefits for the brain. Here are the merits of some more popular choices:

  ✔ **Gingko biloba.** Gingko biloba is a Chinese herb commonly used to enhance memory. You can find Chinese herbal stores in most shopping centres. But does Gingko biloba really deliver in improving your memory? The largest randomised clinical trial, which included over 3,000 elderly adults (70 to 95 years old), investigated the claim that Gingko biloba can improve cognitive functions. Researchers gave these adults a dose of Gingko biloba, or a placebo, twice a day. However, the study, which was conducted in six medical centres across the United States, found no benefits of Gingko biloba on reducing cognitive decline. Gingko biloba didn't reduce the incidence of Alzheimer's, dementia, or even general cognitive skills such as memory, language, attention, or visual-spatial skills. This pattern was true regardless of the age, sex, race, and educational level of the adults – none of this mattered.

The bottom line is that no evidence proves that Gingko biloba lives up to its great expectations – it doesn't improve memory. In fact, taking Gingko biloba may increase the risk of a stroke, and it's been linked to bleeding-related complications.

✔ **Ginseng.** Ginseng is a root herb that's often sold dried, either whole or in slices. Although ginseng has a number of uses, ranging from treating type 2 diabetes to sex dysfunction in men, people most commonly take it as a means to cope with stress. The evidence on whether ginseng can actually improve your brain is limited to animal research. To date, no strong research studies demonstrate the clear benefits of ginseng on the brain. Also bear in mind that Siberian ginseng is sometimes marketed as ginseng. However, Siberian ginseng is a different plant product and there have been far fewer studies on the benefits, if any, of Siberian ginseng on the brain.

✔ **Gotu Kola.** Gotu Kola, like Gingko biloba, has roots in ancient traditional medicines. Ayurvedic and traditional Chinese medicine use Gotu Kola to alleviate symptoms of anxiety and depression. Some evidence suggests that Gotu Kola can minimise these feelings of anxiety and reduce tension and irritability. In healthy adults Gotu Kola was effective in reducing anxiety levels. However, more research is needed to know whether Gotu Kola can also be effective in diminishing feelings of anxiety and irritability in those with anxiety disorders.

There can be serious side effects in mixing herbal treatments with prescribed medication, so it's most important to check with, and notify, your physician if you're taking herbal products. Also, if you do take these herbal supplements, be sure to buy them from a reputable and trusted source.

# Chapter 14

# Building Up Mind/Body Fitness

*In This Chapter*

▶ Working out for your brain

▶ Resting your brain to make the day count

*I*n this chapter I discuss two very different approaches to keeping your brain healthy. In the first part I provide tips on how moving your body keeps your brain active as well. In the second part I look at how resting your body keeps your brain in balance to help it perform at its optimum level.

## Moving Your Body to Keep Your Brain Healthy

The physical benefits of exercise are often more obvious than the cognitive benefits. You can easily see your body looking better and feel healthier. Exercise's benefits to your brain may be harder to notice, but they do exist, from finding it easier to absorb new information to preserving your memory as you get older.

### Comparing running and yoga

You have so many choices when it comes to exercising. Your local gym may present many options when it comes to exercise classes, some of which you may never even have heard of! So is it better to go for the Salsa Beat, Boxercise, or just stick with the treadmill?

## Countering radiation's effects

Exercise is great for the healthy individual, but can exercise counter the effects of radiation treatment on the brain? The answer is 'yes'!

When children receive radiation treatment for tumours in the brain, one unfortunate side effect that sometimes occurs is learning and memory difficulties later in life. Behavioural problems, such as attention-deficit hyperactivity disorder (ADHD), can also show up. So what happens to the brain during radiation treatment? The treatment kills brain stem cells that are in the *hippocampus*, the part of the brain linked with memory and learning.

A study looking at this issue found that exercise resulted in 50 per cent more stem cells in those who exercised compared to those who didn't. These new cells functioned really well. The take-home message is that exercise can regenerate parts of the brain that are damaged and lead to new stem cells that result in enhanced memory and learning.

The following list offers advice on what the research shows works best:

- ✔ **Running counts more.** Studies have confirmed that aerobic activity leads to more benefits from your brain than activities that focus on concentration or toning, like meditation and yoga (see Chapter 10 for more on these topics). As people grow older, the human brain begins to lose tissue, which results in deterioration of cognitive skills. Aerobic exercise is one clear way to delay and in some cases even reverse the effects that age and injury have on the brain.

- ✔ **Age matters.** Studies have found that exercise in young adults improves memory when learning new things. Exercise acts to consolidate the new and incoming information. As you get older and perhaps exercise less, you supplement physical activities with cognitive ones (see Chapters 15 to 17). But keeping up with exercise as you get older is crucial. You may notice changes to your memory, and exercise is key to preserving your ability to recall. Even 20 to 30 minutes each day can prevent memory decline over time.

- ✔ **Keep it beating.** The key to picking an exercise activity for brain reasons is to keep your heart rate up for the duration of the activity. For this *aerobic activity* you need to use oxygen to create energy. Aerobic activities include keeping your heartbeat constant throughout the activity, rather than at short bursts. Examples include running, cycling, and swimming. If you want to boost your brain power, get started on aerobic exercise.

In contrast, anaerobic activity is where your body creates energy without oxygen, for example by playing racquetball, tennis, or weight lifting, where you use short bursts of energy.

The recommended amount of aerobic exercise varies from 20 minutes a day to 60 minutes a day. Examples of aerobic activities include walking, running, swimming, and cycling.

## Finding your ideal level

The key to maximising your aerobic activity for your brain is to make sure that when you exercise you reach within 60 to 90 per cent of your maximum heart rate. Here's a breakdown of the different heart rate levels:

- ✔ **50–60 per cent of maximum heart rate.** This is the easy stuff – what your heart rate does during a warm up or a light stretching programme.

- ✔ **60–70 per cent of maximum heart rate.** This is known as the *Fat Burning Zone*. But based on the scientific research I discuss in this chapter, I call it the *Brain Booster Zone*.

---

## The ADHD solution?

ADHD is often characterised by behaviour problems, such as hyperactivity and an inability to focus on one task at a time. With prevalence rates on the rise, more and more people are looking for alternative ways to manage their symptoms on a daily basis. One way that's growing in popularity is exercise – in fact, some people have even called it 'nature's alternative to methylphenidate' (the medication used to treat the symptoms of ADHD).

You may have heard of Michael Phelps, the Olympian swimmer who won a whopping eight gold medals in a single Olympics, more than any other Olympian. Phelps was diagnosed with ADHD when he was younger, and to help him direct his surplus energy his mother enrolled him in swimming classes. It wasn't long before his coach spotted his talent and he set his first national (USA) record by the time he was 10. And the rest, as they say, is sporting history. Many people say that Phelps's ADHD gave him a huge reserve of energy, and exercising at the level that he did allowed him to overcome many of the behaviour problems associated with ADHD.

Phelps was on medication for ADHD, but the structure and rigorous nature of his training allowed him – after consultation with his family doctor – to stop taking medication.

Scientific research supports the view that exercise has tremendous effects on behaviour. School children who ran around for 15 to 45 minutes before class reduced their hyperactive behaviour by 50 per cent when they came back to class. And these effects lasted up to four hours after the exercise. Good news for any classroom teacher of unruly students.

> ✔ **70–80 per cent of maximum heart rate.** Also great for your brain.
>
> ✔ **80–90 per cent of maximum heart rate.** At this level you have the additional bonus of getting your body to combat tiredness and lethargy during the day.

So how can you calculate your target heart rate? Simple – just subtract your age from 220 to find out what your heart rate should be to achieve the best results for your brain.

## Feeling good from exercise

Exercise is also great for your mental health. It doesn't just leave you feeling good, but it can also improve feelings of depression and anxiety (see Chapter 9 for more on how to improve your mental health).

*Plasticity* or *neuroplasticity* is the way the brain can change throughout your life by forming new connections between brain cells, which are called *neurons*. Most of the change occurs during infancy and childhood when the brain is learning and growing the most. But the brain can also change after an injury that's damaged some part of its functioning. More recently, science has also discovered that the brain is 'plastic', even in adulthood. Whenever you're learning something new, your brain changes to adapt to this new information (see Chapter 7 for how this happens with taxi drivers). Exercise also plays a role in brain cell (neuron) growth in the hippocampus of adults.

Schizophrenia is associated with smaller brain volume, particularly in the hippocampus, which is associated with learning and memory (see Chapter 7). Recent clinical trials have demonstrated that physical exercise can also help increase the volume of the hippocampus in adults with schizophrenia. But the type of exercise made all the difference. Patients who were playing table football, which just enhances concentration and coordination but not fitness levels, didn't increase their brain volume by much at all. In contrast, those who cycled three times a week for 30 minutes increased their brain volume 12 times more than the table football group. This exciting research demonstrates that aerobic activity can make a big difference to adults struggling with difficulties like schizophrenia.

It's not just people with schizophrenia who struggle with memory loss associated with the hippocampus. As people grow older the brain cell growth in the hippocampus decreases, which can also contribute to memory loss. However, exercise can also reverse these effects related to aging. How does exercise do this? It restores a brain chemical that encourages the production of new brain stem cells. When the hippocampus isn't producing brain stem cells, this leads to memory loss and difficulty in absorbing new information. Exercise, however, promotes the production of various chemicals in the brain responsible for new brain cells in the hippocampus.

If you're feeling low, exercise can change your mental health. For one study researchers tested a group of people for their mood – for example, did they feel depressed, or did they feel happy? Over half of the participants were depressed. The participants then did aerobics for one hour. The group of people experiencing depression reported significant changes after the exercise – they no longer felt stressed and tense, their anger levels dropped, and they even felt more energetic after the workout.

Exercise also improves the mental health of older adults. In another study researchers asked a group of 50-year-olds diagnosed with depression to exercise for four months. The participants reported big improvements in their mood at the end of the programme, and they continued to feel good even six months after the exercise programme ended. In fact, their mental health was much better than those who were taking anti-depressants. I'm not suggesting that you throw away any prescribed medication; however, according to strong evidence, if you're feeling low, don't head for the alcohol cabinet. Instead, throw on a good pair of shoes and go for a walk.

# Getting Started On an Exercise Programme

If you've been reading this chapter from the beginning, I hope by now you're convinced of the benefits of exercising. But everyone has days when they look at the rain clouds outside, and it seems so much easier just to stay indoors or go back to bed. So if you're having trouble getting started on an exercise programme, here are some lifelines to get you moving.

✔ **Phone a friend.** Exercising with a friend can increase your motivation. I remember when I was taking an exercise class in the middle of winter. Even though the class was at six in the evening, the dark and cold winter nights always made me wish I wasn't going. However, I never missed a class! The secret? It wasn't my fantastic will power – it was the fact that a friend went to every class with me. I didn't want to be the one to call and cancel. So if you want to stick with your exercise programme the first thing to do is find someone you know who'll go with you. If you can't persuade anyone then join a club. I know someone who joined a running club and goes every week because he doesn't want to be the only one who doesn't show up.

✔ **Go 50/50.** With so many choices of activities to do it's sometimes easier not to do any of them! Think about what you like to do before you even look up the list of classes at your local gym. After you've thought about your own preferences, look right away to see whether the gym offers these choices. This helps you avoid feeling overwhelmed. Narrow your choices by picking just two things and remember that activities that involve aerobic activities are better for your brain.

Some people prefer to work out at home. If this sounds like you, you have a host of great exercise DVDs and videos to choose from, so don't use the weather as an excuse not to exercise! Pick a DVD that you enjoy and get started. If you're buying the DVD online, you can often read reviews from other people, which can help you to select one that best suits your own interests.

✔ **Ask the audience.** As with most things, fad exercises are unlikely to provide long-term benefits. Some activities just last the distance for a reason – they actually work! So when you're deciding what to do to get your heart rate up, find out what the most popular classes are at your local gym. Then sign up as quickly as you can! If you don't enjoy classes and prefer to use the exercise machines, find out which machines are most used and stake out your place early.

If that just isn't enough to get you out of the armchair and exercising, take on board these additional tips and encouragements to remind you to get moving:

✔ **Remind yourself how good you'll feel afterwards.** Exercising offers a great boost to the brain – your brain releases *endorphins* – a chemical that promotes that 'feel-good' sensation – when you exercise. So the next time you need motivation for your workout, whether it's a brisk walk in the park or a run around your neighbourhood, remind yourself of how good you felt the last time you went.

✔ **Set a goal for yourself.** Some people find that having a goal to work towards can make a big difference. Maybe you can sign up for a 5-kilometre run or walk. Having a goal like this in sight can make it easier for you to motivate yourself to get moving.

If you don't like walking or running, sign up for an exercise class and set goals for yourself there. Maybe you're at level 1 and you want to be able to move up to level 2. You can even set targets for yourself if you're using an exercise DVD at home, or a computer-related exercise game. Most DVDs and exercise games have different levels, so just set yourself a time frame for when you hope to move up to the next level.

✔ **Tell other people what you're doing.** Make sure that your friends and family know about the goal you've set for yourself. This way if you feel like slacking off, they can help to keep you accountable.

✔ **Reward yourself.** When you reach your goal, give yourself a treat. And no, I don't mean chocolate! Your reward may be something small like a new book you've been waiting to read or something more extravagant, like a pampering weekend. Whatever you decide, having something to look forward to when you reach your goal offers an extra incentive for you to get there.

# Resting Your Brain

Sleep is the one thing everyone can always use more of, but the reality is that between juggling all their different responsibilities, people seldom get that magic eight hours a night. Now you can 'rest' assured that it doesn't matter. If you want to boost your brain power, this section provides tips to help.

Sleep has five stages. Here's a quick overview of what happens at each stage:

✔ **Stage 1.** In Stage 1 sleep is at the light stage and you find yourself drifting in and out of sleep and easily woken up. Sudden muscle contractions aren't uncommon in this stage, which can cause you to jump or get startled when someone tries to wake you. Think of the last time you fell asleep on a plane. You were probably only at Stage 1 in your sleep cycle when the stewardess woke you up to ask whether you wanted something to eat!

✔ **Stage 2.** In Stage 2 eye movements stop and brain waves become slower. You spend about 50 per cent of your sleep cycle in this stage, in which your *brain waves* (which measure your brain activity) become slower.

✔ **Stages 3 and 4.** Stages 3 and 4 are known as *deep sleep.* Waking someone up during these stages is very difficult, and when you try the person is often disorientated and groggy for a few minutes. These two stages are critical times for your brain to refresh itself.

✔ **Stage 5.** Stage 5 is *REM* (rapid eye movement), which comes at the end of sleep. Adults usually only spend about 20 per cent of their sleep cycle at the REM stage, and the bulk of sleep time in stage 2 (50 per cent). Babies, however, spend more than half their sleep cycle in the REM stage. Psychologists speculate that REM sleep is critical for learning because the brain consolidates learning by transferring it into long-term memory during this time.

Why is it so hard to remember that early morning phone conversation? Because brain activity is slower during some sleep stages, your brain 'erases' events if you were asleep, awoken, and then fall back asleep again. So if you're prone to receiving important calls in the middle of the night, keep a notebook and pen by your bedside to scribble down the important message because without that, you won't remember the message in the morning.

## Getting better rest

If you're feeling sleep-deprived, take on board these few tips to maximise your zzzs:

✔ **Pass on the liqueur.** Contrary to what you may think, alcohol doesn't help you sleep better. In fact, alcohol consumption before bed prevents you from reaching deep sleep, which means that your brain can't refresh itself in time for the following day. Habits develop early, and research found that alcohol abuse during teenage years leads to sleep problems later in life.

✔ **Bring back the siesta.** Europeans have the right idea with their midday snoozes. And now science is on their side. People who take 90 minute naps during the day are much better at performing cognitive tasks in the evening than those who haven't had a nap. Some have described the effect of naps on the brain like clearing your email inbox when it's full. Naps allow your brain to clear out what it doesn't need to make room for important incoming information. Without sleep, your brain store registers as 'full' and has a hard time taking in new information.

✔ **Show me the light.** Frequent travellers sometimes use light therapy to help people recover from jet lag. Even a few milliseconds of extremely bright light can significantly improve alertness and brain functioning. You can also see benefits of sunlight on your brain – so make sure that you spend at least 15 minutes each day in sunlight.

## Don't get up yet, lazy bones

Teenagers have a reputation for sleeping in late in the morning, as any parent trying to rush them off to school knows well. And usually, despite your best efforts, they don't plan on changing anything. Well, now science is on their side. Studies have found that at the onset of puberty teenagers develop a delayed sleep pattern known as a *two-hour sleep-wake phase.* This simply means that that due to their body's changing needs they need to go to sleep later at night and need more sleep in the morning. Teenagers still only need about nine hours of sleep each night; they just need it at different times.

So how does this different sleep pattern affect the teenage brain? In a recent study one high school decided to delay the start time to allow their students to get extra sleep in the morning. The teenagers were more alert and reported feeling less irritated during the day. Their mental health also improved and fewer students reported feeling depressed. Fewer students skipped class, which meant that opportunities for learning were better. The study was considered a success by the school and the students, and the late start for the school is now a permanent fixture. So the next time you have trouble getting your teenager out of bed, remember she's building her brain with her sleep patterns.

✔ **Maximise productivity.** Find the time of the day when you work best and maximise your time. If you're most productive in the morning, turn off all other distractions and use that time to swot up on what you need to do. If you work best in the morning, resist the urge to read the news or surf the web. Instead, focus on the urgent activities that you need to accomplish. That way, you can enjoy relaxing.

## *Sleeping your way to a better brain*

Don't underestimate the power of sleep for your brain. Sleeping is a time for more than just 'resting your eyes'.

Your brain needs sleep so your nervous system can work efficiently. A lack of sleep leads to impaired memory skills and poor judgement. Even simple tasks like solving a maths problem become difficult when you lack sleep. During sleep your brain has a chance to shut down the 'circuits' that were busy working during the day and allows them to recharge and refresh. A lack of sleep means that your brain neurons or circuits start losing energy and underperform. You've probably experienced this if you've had to work late for an extended period.

Sleep is critical for children. They use this time not only to grow physically, but also to develop brain building blocks crucial for decision-making. Studies have found that children who get less sleep have more behavioural problems. This explains why the over-tired child seems extra emotional or can't stop complaining. The lack of sleep means that the child can't moderate her emotions or control her behaviour very well and can act in an unruly manner.

Bear in mind these tips for making sure that your beauty sleep is really refreshing your brain:

- **Match your sleep with your age.** How much sleep is enough? The answer depends on your age. Babies need around 16 hours a day, and adults need around 8 hours. Pregnant women, especially in the first trimester, need a few more hours. As you get older, you need less sleep.

  But it's not just the number of hours that's important; the pattern of sleep is also crucial. For example, teenagers need more sleep in the morning for their brain to function effectively (see the sidebar 'Don't get up yet, lazy bones').

  As people get older, they need less sleep. However, studies have found that older people are still able to perform well on different cognitive tasks that involve memory and attention. In elderly populations the brain compensates for the lack of sleep by using other mechanisms that result in a state of *hyperarousal*. Hyperarousal is similar to a mild form of stress and can boost the brain's performance.

- **Morning light, brain is bright.** The part of the brain that controls emotions, social skills, and decision-making shuts down during deep sleep. When you're awake, you're able to be more rational and logical in both professional and personal relationships. So avoid making major decisions when you're tired – you'll almost certainly regret them after a good night's sleep.

- **Keep it moderate.** The temperature, that is. If your room is too cold or too hot, it can disrupt your sleep cycle. If you're going to be outside in very hot or cold temperatures, be aware that your body can't regulate its temperature during REM sleep. This means that your sleep can easily be disrupted by the temperatures and you won't reach REM sleep. When this happens, your body can lose its sleep cycle during your next bedtime. So if you're planning outdoor activities with temperature drops, be sure to dress appropriately, especially at night. Your brain will thank you.

- **Stick to a schedule.** Your brain will also thank you for going to bed at the same time everyday. It helps your sleep schedule. You may find that when you sleep in during the weekend you feel more lethargic and tired despite getting more sleep. That's because your body is used to the schedule. So if you're going to have a late night, plan it on Saturday and not on Sunday. Otherwise, you throw off your sleep schedule for Monday.

✔ **Move it.** You can't use the old excuse that you're too tired to exercise. Scientists have discovered that even 15 minutes a day can make a big difference to your sleep cycle. Exercise helps you get REM sleep and feel more awake during the day. But it's not just any exercise that does the trick. You need to do some cardiovascular activity that gets your heart pumping for at least 20 minutes. Nothing, not even yoga or stretches, matches the sleep-enhancing benefits of such a workout. However, remember not to exercise too vigorously close to bedtime, because you'll raise your body temperature, which makes falling asleep more difficult. Read more about exercising for your brain in the section 'Comparing running and yoga', earlier in this chapter.

If you're not getting enough sleep, don't think that your brain will adjust. It won't. Your brain develops a 'deficit', or 'sleep debt', and you need to catch up in order to function well. The optimum amount of sleep that an adult needs varies from person to person. Just because your friend can function well on six hours a night doesn't mean that you can too. You may be able to last for a few days by 'burning the candle at both ends', but eventually you'll notice a big drop in your everyday activities, from driving to organising meetings, to holding conversations.

REM sleep stimulates the brain regions you use in learning. This stage is especially important for babies, which is why they spend twice as much time in REM sleep compared to adults. But don't think that REM sleep isn't important for you too. Studies have found that adults learn new skills best after REM sleep. When adults are deprived of REM sleep, they're not able to master new skills. Keep that thought in mind the next time you want to stay up late before an exam at school or an important presentation at work.

_Neurotransmitter signals_ – chemical messengers that run between different brain cells – in the brain affect sleep patterns. What can affect these signals? For starters, the food you eat can make a big difference to these neurotransmitter signals. For example, whole grains and leafy green vegetables work to promote sleep, and milk is an old remedy for insomnia. Milk contains tryptophan – an amino acid – that gets converted to serotonin, which is one of the neurotransmitters that regulate sleep.

# While you were sleeping

You may have heard of the amazing story of American Terry Wallis – the man who slept for 19 years. Terry was in a car accident when he was 19 years old and as a result was in a coma. He then moved into a minimally conscious state, in which he remained for almost 20 years!

Then one day he woke up. His first question to the nurse was, 'Who is that?' He didn't recognise his mother and still thought he was 19 years old. When asked who the US president was he replied that it was Ronald Reagan, because he was still stuck in 1984, the year of his accident.

About half the people who sustain head injuries and end up in a coma are able to recover some awareness and cognitive functioning. However, Terry showed very little improvement in the first year after waking from his coma. Although his parents took him home every other week and talked to him regularly, he didn't respond. Eventually, the doctors pronounced him to be in a persistent vegetative state with little chance of recovery.

And then Terry proved them all wrong. He eventually came round and started using one-word utterances like *Pepsi* and *dad* to communicate what he wanted. He could even recognise his daughter, who was 6 weeks old at the time of his crash. His first words to her were, 'You are beautiful.'

What happened to Terry's brain while he was in a coma? Using cutting-edge scientific technology, doctors were able to understand more about Terry's brain. They found evidence of new growth in two key areas in his brain. His cerebellum, which is linked with motor control, was still developing. This new growth allowed him to regain his strength in his arms and legs. The doctors also found new growth at the back of his brain, which is linked with conscious awareness. Terry Wallis is walking evidence of the power of the brain to heal itself even after traumatic head injury.

Other foods and stimulants can interfere with these signals. Caffeine is an easy one – it stimulates parts of the brain and keeps you awake. Diet pills and some decongestants (those meant for using during the day) have the same effect on sleep patterns, as does smoking. Sleep patterns of smokers are also affected because they usually wake up after four hours due to nicotine withdrawals.

Alcohol has the opposite effect – it induces sleep. But hold off before you reach for the extra glass of wine. Although alcohol does trigger sleep, it's only the light stage of sleep, which means that the slightest noise can easily wake you. Your brain needs REM sleep to restore itself but alcohol before bed doesn't allow sleep patterns to reach this stage. In other words, by drinking alcohol as a night-cap, you're robbing your brain of the best sleep it needs.

Sleep deprivation has serious consequences. Studies have found that people who are sleep-deprived drive as poorly as those who are over the legal limit in alcohol. If you're not getting enough sleep, this can also magnify the effect of alcohol on your body. This means that when you have a pint of beer when you're tired, you feel the effects much more than if you were well-rested.

 Are people in a coma just asleep? Their brain patterns are very different – for example, they don't produce the same complex patterns that healthy people do while asleep. Brain patterns of people in comas are very slow, and in some cases, can be difficult to detect.

# Part V

# Game On! Brain Training Games to Play at Home

## The 5th Wave

By Rich Tennant

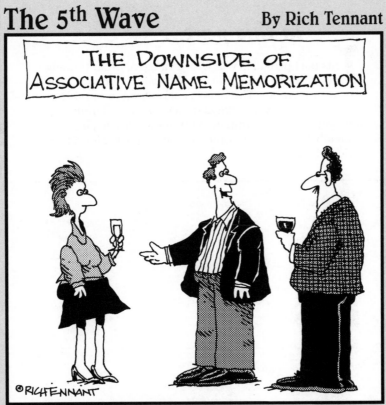

THE DOWNSIDE OF ASSOCIATIVE NAME MEMORIZATION

"John nose hairs, I'd like you to meet Barbara parrot face."

## In this part...

*T*his part provides you with a range of brain training activities to train your verbal brain, your spatial brain, and your memory. The part is guaranteed to provide you with fun and engaging ways to make a big difference in how you use your brain in everyday situations, from remembering your shopping list to preparing for a presentation at work.

# Chapter 15

# Verbal Brain Games

. . . . . . . . . . . . . . . . . . . . . . . . . . . . . . . . . . . . . .

## *In This Chapter*

▶ Getting wordy over word puzzles
▶ Cracking the codes on crossword puzzles

. . . . . . . . . . . . . . . . . . . . . . . . . . . . . . . . . . . . . .

*E*ver heard of something called 'cognitive reserve'? Well, the idea of *cognitive reserve* has recently become a buzz word in the scientific community. This theory essentially says that people who have a larger reserve of neurons and stronger cognitive abilities can tolerate some brain deterioration without showing symptoms. In other words, the more you use your brain, the greater your chances of avoiding symptoms of memory loss.

This chapter provides verbal brain games to get you started on building up your very own cognitive reserve.

## *Scrambling Words*

Some people adore puzzles that allow them to play with words: crosswords, logic puzzles, riddles, word searches, word scrambles, and so on. They just seem to have the knack of solving them. Others don't have the knack at all, and wouldn't recognise it if it smacked them in the forehead.

So, how do you get the knack? If you want to be able to look a puzzle squarely in the face and say, 'You're not keeping me awake tonight!' what can you do (other than keep the answers handy)?

Many people start working on puzzles in school, when teachers get their pupils to take on puzzles that reinforced spelling, reading, science, or other lessons of the day. Chances are you've been familiar with the structure of most of these puzzles for a long time, and you've probably had at least some experience working them.

But that doesn't necessarily mean you're comfortable with them. In fact, you may feel downright nervous when you sit down to work a crossword these days. After all, what better way is there to test how much knowledge you've accumulated – and retained – over the years? And what better way to feel like a complete dipstick than to find yourself staring blankly at clue after clue?

Maybe you've long avoided some of these puzzles precisely because they point out how much you don't know. And maybe you're now ready to overcome your fears. Plus, they're a lot of fun – after you get past the fear and frustration.

## *Getting a feel for different types of word scrambles*

You can play word scramble puzzles in various ways.

You look at a group of letters placed in a random order and rearrange them into one word, using every letter. The words that you're rearranging may be rather short – between five and eight characters. For example, unscramble the capitalised word to solve this riddle:

Where a sauce may THICKEN: _ _ _ _ _ _ _

The answer to this riddle, by the way, is *kitchen*. Unscrambling words of this length isn't usually very difficult (although I won't dare suggest that you'll never get stuck!). The difficulty increases along with the number of letters and words involved. For example, try to solve this one:

Where's a good place to see a SCHOOL MASTER? _ _ _ _ _ _ _ _ _ _ _ _

The answer is *the classroom*.

After you solve several word scrambles like these two examples, you then take a second step. You circle certain characters in those words, and by using only the circled letters, you solve one more scramble: you rearrange the letters to create a word or phrase that answers a clue given by the puzzle constructor.

In this step, you're likely to be dealing with quite a few characters, and you're often creating more than one word. As with the *kitchen* and *the classroom* examples, the puzzle constructor usually provides blanks that show how many words are in the solution and how many characters are in each.

Another word scramble puzzle is to look at a group of letters and try to create as many words as possible from them. You don't have to use every letter in every word you create. For example, if you have eight letters, you can create words with three letters, four letters, and so on. The goal is to make as many words as possible, and the puzzle constructor may tell you how many words you're aiming for. The puzzle constructor may also set certain rules, such as no two-letter words.

## Being strategic

The strategies for approaching word scrambles are pretty straightforward:

- ✔ If you're working on a series of jumbled words, look at each one in turn to see if any words jump out at you. You'll be amazed by how quickly you can solve some scrambles; the mind seems built for this type of task.

- ✔ When an answer doesn't jump out at you, try writing the letters in a different order. Don't worry about creating a word right away – just putting the letters in a new order may trigger that 'Aha!' moment you're looking for.

- ✔ If the 'Aha!' remains elusive, try grouping together letters in what seems to be a logical way. Consider how many vowels you have; if you have twice as many consonants as vowels, chances are the word begins with a consonant. Try putting together common groupings such as *ing, sh* or *th*.

  Keep rearranging letters for as long as it takes to find what you're looking for. You can even put the letters randomly in a circle to help you view the letters differently. Eventually, you'll stumble upon a combination that makes sense.

- ✔ If you're playing the type of scramble where you make as many words as you can out of a group of letters, be sure to look for words that you can pull directly from within the words you've already created. For example, if you've written down *player*, be sure to also write down *play, lay,* and *layer.* You can also write down *pay, per, year, reap,* and so on, but the point is to notice the words that you've already spelled out, in order, within the longer words you've created – they're your easiest finds.

## Giving word scrambles a try

Unscramble the capitalised word(s) in quotations to solve the riddles.

### Easy

**Puzzle 1**
_____

What some feel ELVIS does? _ _ _ _ _

**Puzzle 2**
_____

What some ACTORS hate to do? _ _ -_ _ _ _

**Puzzle 3**
_____

What mishandling ROSES can lead to? _ _ _ _ _

**Puzzle 4**
_____

How a RESCUE can make the saved person feel? _ _ _ _ _ _

### Tricky

**Puzzle 5**
_____

Easy thing to do when you're SILENT? _ _ _ _ _ _

**Puzzle 6**
_____

What THE EYES do? _ _ _ _ _ _ _

**Puzzle 7**
_____

What THE IRS thinks your money is? _ _ _ _ _ _

**Puzzle 8**
_____

What courtroom figures in ROBES are? _ _ _ _ _

**Puzzle 9**
_____

Simple thing to do with a STIPEND? _ _ _ _ _ _ _

**Puzzle 10**
_____

While a teacher may be TEACHING, a student may be? _ _ _ _ _ _ _ _

**Puzzle 11**

Where a sauce may THICKEN _ _ _ _ _ _ _

## Tough
**Puzzle 12**

Option for those with BAD CREDIT? _ _ _ _ _ _ _ _ _

**Puzzle 13**

This occurs when something is PAST DUE? _ _ _ _ ' _ _ _

**Puzzle 14**

Where's a good place to see a SCHOOL MASTER? _ _ _ _ _ _ _ _ _ _ _ _

## Treacherous, not tough
**Puzzle 15**

What illegal auto RACES CAN RUIN? _ _ _ _ _ _ _ _ _ _ _ _

**Puzzle 16**

What THE DETECTIVES do? _ _ _ _ _ _ _ _ _ _ _ _

**Puzzle 17**

What's TWELVE PLUS ONE? _ _ _ _ _ _ _ _ _ _ _ _

## Treacherous
**Puzzle 18**

What's HOTTER IN DEGREES? _ _ _ _ _ _ _ _ _ _ _ _ _ _

**Puzzle 19**

PAYMENT RECEIVED! _ _ _ _ _ _ _ _ _ _ _ _ _ _

**Puzzle 20**

Many people leave SLOT MACHINES with? _ _ _ _ _ _ _ _ _ _ ' _ _

**Puzzle 21**

What a CURE FOR BALD MALES may be? _ _ _ _ _ _ _ _ _ _ _ _ _ _ _

**Puzzle 22**

One in a group of NOTIONS WE RARELY USE? _ _ _ _ _ _ _ _ ' _ _ _ _ _ _ _ _ _

# Relaxing with Word Searches

As with crossword puzzles, you were probably introduced to word searches early in life. Most people do word searches them in primary school to reinforce their spelling and vocabulary lessons.

In case you've never seen one before, a word search is simply a grid of letters – in a square or rectangular shape – that contains hidden words. Your goal is to find and circle the words, which may appear horizontally, vertically,` or diagonally within the grid. Some words may be written backwards. Some compilers construct word searches around a central theme, which means all the words you find relate to one topic.

## Being strategic

The thing I love about word searches is they're really low stress. If a word list is provided, I guarantee you can complete the search – no matter how large the grid or how many words you're looking for. How often in life do you get the satisfaction of knowing you're going to get the right answers? That fact, in itself, makes working word searches fun. Plus, they're great puzzles for increasing your concentration and blocking out the world for a while.

## *Trying your hand at word searches*

Where to begin with word searches? Here are my suggestions:

✔ Use a pencil rather than a pen. Some people will disagree with me, insisting that working in pen is the only way to go. But until you get truly comfortable at working these puzzles, don't give yourself a reason to stress about mistakes!

✔ Read through the words one by one and find those that seem obvious. Even in the toughest puzzle, you're likely to find at least one or two words immediately.

✔ After you circle the easy answers, go back and try your hand at the tougher ones.

Take your time with this step, and don't get frustrated if answers don't jump to mind immediately. You may be still getting familiar with doing this type of word puzzle.

*Easy*

```
Y M C W J E Z Q K O O H T A E M Q O E U V
K E E T M A N A G E M E N T P F I P A L M
I C V U F O X T U P U A X Q V O H T J L X
P N J N D I D T N A D N E T T A V S T E C
E A X L O V L U F L D H G D Z V T S T T O
G D O F E C M Z J D A V E P H A O M S A M
R I X Y M J V B R S J L R Y F H Q J I I M
A U I E K L L I S O I L I F S G L A F C A
H G H W S B M I B V O C E U H N N X J O N
C I W R X Q S H E A W R P W O R K E R S D
A I E F K T O R C N E P M M J Q A X Y S T
Q V G T A L G I T H O M Q U W P Q T Z A H
T Y Y N D L E R C R E S L A B O U R E R B
I G T E A K B J T U I U E N U X C G B X Q
L R R D I A O K G D W D J Y H O W X D O L
D N A H D B Y A E F G Z G E T K G W J A X
L Z X I E J E K D F N B L E N Y O L U W L
E Z C T I L I O X F G P Y H J T S N K M A
Q Q U E L C G V N F E B F V E D A R M O C
W Z K O K Y X K Q R D E R I H M O J D W B
C L C K S Y Q P F R E E Y O L P M E S Q K
```

**Puzzle 23**

| | | |
|---|---|---|
| AIDE | EMPLOYEE | MANUAL |
| ASSISTANT | FIST | MEATHOOK |
| ASSOCIATE | GUIDANCE | MITT |
| ATTENDANT | HAND | PALM |
| CHARGE | HELPER | SIDEKICK |
| COLLEAGUE | HIRED | STAFFER |
| COMMAND | JOBHOLDER | SUPPORT |
| COMRADE | LABOURER | WORKER |
| CONVEY | LIFT | |
| DELIVER | MANAGEMENT | |

*Tough*

```
M D N A E Z B A L M O E P I U U T W B I Y
X R O O I K A N L J B C F X A E C Y L A T
E V L J Y N I E E C L W A E W S A D G S Y
V E T I Q A J O T K I F D R J I X N P P X
O S R N M S L P X T G Z S O D R E I C T G
E N M C A P E B C N A L P C M O L O T P C
A K U C E R O U C T T E B T F H G J G N W
K T A Q B D R S K M E P R A F T P N H D K
P P N M H T I A E M Z M K J L U J E L W L
L Y H I S E J V W U L O F L S A T V R Y L
N T D N O A A L H S P C I U U Q H E L B E
E U I S L P S M L I O O U V M K D K I T E
G D M E E X P Y C F Z F N P M R D N A R F
R R E R F G B A Z G P S X E O Z B N I A D
A F G N O P U T C I L F N I N U G U C R N
H E B I R C S E R P M I O U F I Q L I I A
C G B R C F Z N L K J A J F S E V V J R M
F R Y G E V W A G U O K O E R E W U Y D E
E R U J D A C C O H R O D L E T A T C I D
A S S I G N K T L B N O U U F K A D W X E
U Y C T C E R I D H V G D N A M M O C S Z
```

**Puzzle 24**

| | | |
|---|---|---|
| ADJURE | DIRECT | OBLIGATE |
| APPOINT | ENACT | ORDER |
| ASSIGN | ENJOIN | PRESCRIBE |
| AUTHORISE | EXACT | REQUIRE |
| CHARGE | FORCE | RULE |
| COMMAND | GIVEORDERS | SUBPOENA |
| COMPEL | IMPOSEUPON | SUMMON |
| DECREE | INFLICTUPON | TELL |
| DEMAND | INSTRUCT | WARRANT |
| DESIGNATE | LAYON | |
| DICTATE | MAKE | |

## Treacherous

```
Y D Z S G O E Z T W U W T Z G C C U T H P R Q
Y F I T A R L O L E G A L I S E A D N V W V S
F U I D A O B D E L E G A T E P Y Z A A M B Z
T I F T U O A E T A T I C A P A C F R L M R E
F E H D R L N B M S X K I R H Q D N R I M B T
V L F E V E E O E W O M O M L O O R A D Q Q U
D T L P E H C V C C C V T N P R H C W A C M T
W J W U N X N G O P E U F O T R G L E T I X I
O B P T T I J M E Y S A X J U I Z N H E C M T
Q K F E R A M B Z T N E M U C O D S T L R D S
E J V R U I Y F I L A U Q I W O I J S N F M N
S C Z D S R L I C E N C E E W L U A E M V H O
I U O S T K W S W X R U Z T B A N Z M N B Y C
H I I N X Y G I M R N Y R A D C W P E E D P T
C O L G F C G C E T M K T T T R V Y S S E U I
N G U B I I R T E S P S I I I W Z P I I L I E
A G D W Z Z R Z N Q E B O L G I E Q L R T O E
R V S U Q A T M W O U N W I J R A A A O I F W
F T T R H S D R Z U I I P C Q U S E M H T G Y
X C A C C R E D I T V Q P A X S C L R T N H R
N K B Y S T R I S K C F X F I Q S H O U E E O
E E Y S F U I Z Y W Z N V S T O F P F A H W I
O Y A Q Q P O Q F S N A T F V X O I N M S D Z
```

**Puzzle 25**

| | | |
|---|---|---|
| ACCREDIT | DEPUTE | FRANCHISE |
| APPROVE | DOCUMENT | INVEST |
| ASSIST | ENABLE | LEGALISE |
| AUTHORISE | ENDOW | LICENCE |
| CAPACITATE | ENDUE | OUTFIT |
| CERTIFY | ENTITLE | QUALIFY |
| CHARTER | ENTRUST | RATIFY |
| COMMISSION | EQUIP | SANCTION |
| CONFIRM | ESTABLISH | VALIDATE |
| CONSTITUTE | FACILITATE | WARRANT |
| DELEGATE | FORMALISE | |

# Chapter 16

# Numerical Brain Games

............................................................

............................................................

**S**olving a Sudoku puzzle requires a different kind of mental workout than solving a crossword puzzle or a word scramble. The breadth of your vocabulary and depth of your factual knowledge are pretty much irrelevant here – logic and diligence are your keys to success.

In this chapter, I introduce basic strategies for working a Sudoku puzzle, before then giving you some circular sudoku puzzles to solve.

## Using Logic to Solve Sudoku Puzzles

A basic discipline of Sudoku solving is recognising option groupings. Spotting the relationship of a group of options in one square to another group in another square is fundamental to solving difficult Sudoku puzzles.

## Solving strategies

Here are the basic essentials you need to know to get going with Sudoku:

- The basic Sudoku puzzle is a 9-x-9 grid; it contains nine rows and nine columns, and is divided into nine 3-x-3 grids or boxes. (Tougher puzzles may consist of 12-x-12 or 16-x-16 grids, but I don't include these sizes in this book. I do, however, include some circular or *target* Sudokus, which I discuss at the end of the chapter.)

- Your job is to make sure that each row, column, and 3-x-3 box in the puzzle contains the numbers 1 through to 9. If you do your job correctly, each of these numbers can appear only once in each row, column, and 3-x-3 box.

- Each puzzle has a unique solution; you can't solve a puzzle in more than one way. The difficulty of each puzzle depends on how many numbers are provided and where they're placed.

- When you start a puzzle, your goal is to locate one or more blank cells for which you can identify just one number that 'works'. In other words, you're looking for definite answers – spaces where the numbers provided for a certain row, column, and 3-x-3 box offer enough information for you to eliminate every possibility except one.

  For example, you may find a space in a row that already contains the numbers 2, 5, and 6. The same space may fall in a column that contains 1, 4, and 9. And the 3-x-3 box that houses the space may already have the numbers 3 and 8 in it. When you combine all those clues, you realise that only the number 7 can go in that space. Seven is a definite answer – precisely what you're looking for to get started.

- After you fill in one or more definite answers, you need to go back and consider how those new pieces of information affect the blank spaces you've already considered. Solving one number may be just the step needed to solve another in the same row, column, or 3-x-3 box. ('Aha! I knew that space had to be filled with either a 2 or a 7. Now that I've written 7 elsewhere in this row, my answer has to be 2.')

✔ At some point – sooner rather than later, if the puzzle is a tough one – you're going to run out of obvious answers. Your next step is to start filling in possible answers in each empty space – doing so can help you identify definite answers that have been hiding from you.

You must use a pencil here – you could end up with six or more numbers in a single space! You may even want to make a copy of the puzzle you're working on so you can scratch all over it and write only the definite answers on the original puzzle.

But what do you do after you've identified a bunch of possibilities? What do all these tiny numbers mean, and how do they help you figure out which is correct?

This step of the puzzle is where you have a choice to make: apply strategies such as those I outline in the next section, or start making best guesses and see where each leads you.

Sudoku is a puzzle that you solve with logic alone, so it follows that you need to examine the schemes for solving in a logical way. Finding out about pairs and triplets gives you a good grounding in Sudoku logic and enables you to understand the reasoning behind the more advanced strategies.

## *Trying the puzzles*

I label these puzzles by type and difficulty level. Levels are easy, tough and treacherous, easy being (of course) the easiest puzzles, and treacherous being the most difficult puzzles. When you finish solving all these puzzles, please see the Appendix for the answers. Have fun!

*Easy*

| | | | 3 | 6 | | 9 | 5 |
|---|---|---|---|---|---|---|---|---|
| 3 | | | 9 | | 4 | | 7 | |
| | 9 | 7 | | | | | | |
| | 3 | 1 | 6 | | | | | |
| | | | 2 | | 1 | | | |
| | | | | | 9 | 5 | 4 | |
| | | | | | | 2 | 5 | |
| | 1 | | 4 | | 7 | | | 8 |
| 4 | 6 | | 5 | 9 | | | | |

Puzzle 26

|   |   |   | 6 |   |   | 1 | 7 |   |
|---|---|---|---|---|---|---|---|---|
|   | 8 |   |   | 4 | 1 | 5 |   |   |
|   | 3 |   |   | 2 |   | 4 |   |   |
|   |   |   | 3 | 9 | 4 |   | 2 |   |
|   |   |   |   | 5 |   |   |   |   |
|   | 4 |   | 2 | 6 | 7 |   |   |   |
|   |   | 1 |   | 7 |   |   | 5 |   |
|   |   | 3 | 4 | 1 |   |   | 8 |   |
|   | 2 | 9 |   |   | 3 |   |   |   |

**Puzzle 27**

| | | 1 | 8 | | 6 | 9 | | |
|---|---|---|---|---|---|---|---|---|
| 4 | | 5 | | | | | | |
| | 2 | | 4 | 3 | | | | |
| 9 | | | 7 | 2 | | 5 | | |
| | 8 | | | | | | 1 | |
| | | 2 | | 9 | 8 | | | 6 |
| | | | | 8 | 4 | | 3 | |
| | | | | | | | 8 | 1 |
| | | 4 | 3 | | 2 | 7 | | |

**Puzzle 28**

|   |   | 5 |   | 2 |   | 3 |   |   |
|---|---|---|---|---|---|---|---|---|
| 6 | 3 |   | 4 |   |   |   |   | 9 |
|   |   |   | 3 |   |   |   | 7 |   |
| 2 |   |   |   |   |   | 8 | 9 |   |
| 8 |   | 4 |   |   |   | 6 |   | 1 |
|   | 9 | 3 |   |   |   |   |   | 5 |
|   | 4 |   |   |   | 5 |   |   |   |
| 1 |   |   |   |   | 8 |   | 5 | 4 |
|   |   | 6 |   | 9 |   | 7 |   |   |

**Puzzle 29**

*Tricky*

| | | | | | | | | 8 |
|---|---|---|---|---|---|---|---|---|
| 2 | | 7 | 3 | | | 1 | 9 | |
| | | | 1 | | 5 | | 3 | |
| | | 4 | | 9 | 3 | | | |
| | 6 | | 7 | | 1 | | 2 | |
| | | | 8 | 2 | | 7 | | |
| | 4 | | 2 | | 8 | | | |
| | 1 | 6 | | | 7 | 2 | | 9 |
| 5 | | | | | | | | |

Puzzle 30

|   | 7 |   |   | 5 |   | 1 | 8 |   |
|---|---|---|---|---|---|---|---|---|
|   |   | 4 | 2 |   |   |   |   | 6 |
| 9 | 8 |   |   |   |   |   |   |   |
| 8 | 9 |   | 5 | 2 |   |   |   |   |
| 4 |   |   |   |   |   |   |   | 3 |
|   |   |   |   | 4 | 3 |   | 5 | 8 |
|   |   |   |   |   |   |   | 4 | 1 |
| 3 |   |   |   |   | 5 | 8 |   |   |
|   | 5 | 8 |   | 9 |   |   | 7 |   |

**Puzzle 31**

| 3 |   | 4 |   |   |   | 1 |   | 8 |
|---|---|---|---|---|---|---|---|---|
|   | 6 |   | 9 |   | 3 |   | 2 |   |
|   |   |   |   |   |   |   |   |   |
|   |   | 6 | 8 |   | 2 | 7 |   |   |
| 5 | 2 |   |   |   |   |   | 1 | 6 |
|   |   | 1 | 3 |   | 5 | 9 |   |   |
|   | 3 |   | 7 |   | 1 |   | 5 |   |
| 6 |   | 7 |   |   |   | 2 |   | 3 |

Puzzle 32

| | | | 6 | | | | 1 | 5 |
|---|---|---|---|---|---|---|---|---|
| | | | 4 | | 7 | | 8 | |
| | 6 | | | 9 | | | | 2 |
| | 5 | | 2 | | 1 | | | 7 |
| | | 3 | | | | 9 | | |
| 8 | | | 9 | | 4 | | 3 | |
| 3 | | | | 1 | | | 6 | |
| | 4 | | 7 | | 9 | | | |
| 2 | 1 | | | 4 | | | | |

Puzzle 33

| 6 |   |   | 3 |   | 9 |   |   | 4 |
|---|---|---|---|---|---|---|---|---|
|   |   | 2 |   |   | 1 |   | 5 | 9 |
|   | 9 |   | 7 |   |   | 1 |   |   |
|   | 6 | 4 |   |   |   |   |   | 2 |
|   |   |   |   |   |   |   |   |   |
| 5 |   |   |   |   |   | 4 | 6 |   |
|   |   | 3 |   |   | 2 |   | 4 |   |
| 2 | 1 |   | 4 |   |   | 9 |   |   |
| 4 |   |   | 6 |   | 8 |   |   | 5 |

Puzzle 34

| | 8 | | | 4 | | | 1 | |
|---|---|---|---|---|---|---|---|---|
| | | | 8 | | 1 | | | |
| 7 | | 4 | 6 | | 5 | | | |
| | 6 | 1 | | | | 9 | 4 | |
| 8 | | | | | | | | 1 |
| | 4 | 3 | | | | 5 | 7 | |
| | | | 5 | | 6 | 4 | | 3 |
| | | | 7 | | 4 | | | |
| | 5 | | | 2 | | | 9 | |

Puzzle 35

*Treacherous*

| | | 9 | 4 | 7 | | | 8 | |
|---|---|---|---|---|---|---|---|---|
| 7 | | | | 3 | | | 5 | |
| 8 | | | | | 2 | 6 | | |
| 2 | | | | | 3 | | 1 | |
| | 4 | | | | | | 3 | |
| | 1 | | 5 | | | | | 2 |
| | | 6 | 3 | | | | | 7 |
| | 7 | | | 2 | | | | 8 |
| | 5 | | | 8 | 1 | 3 | | |

Puzzle 36

# Taking Target Practice with Circular Sudoku

If you start getting square eyes from doing regular Sudoku, I can offer some relief in the form of circular Sudoku, sometimes called *target* Sudoku. Think of the puzzle as a big pie cut into eight slices, each slice with four bites. Your goal is to place a number into each bite of pie so that each adjacent slice contains all the numbers from one to eight. Every ring must also contain all the numbers from one to eight.

Here's an important clue: every other pie slice contains the same four numbers. That has to be the case because otherwise, you'd have duplicates in some combination of two adjacent slices. However, the four numbers appear in different orders in the different slices because of the fact that each ring comes into play as well.

As with nine-by-nine grid Sudoku puzzles, you start a target Sudoku by trying to identify definite answers: those blank spaces that can have only one answer based on the numbers the puzzle constructor's provided. Target Sudoku puzzles are a nice change of pace from grid ones and may be a touch easier because you're dealing with fewer spaces to fill.

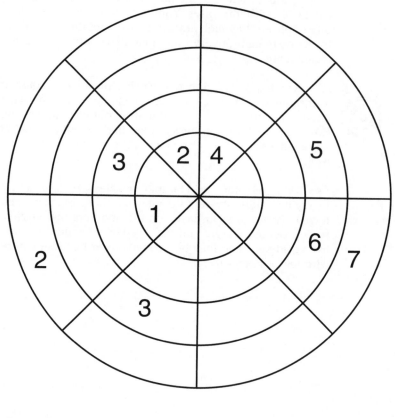

**Puzzle 37**

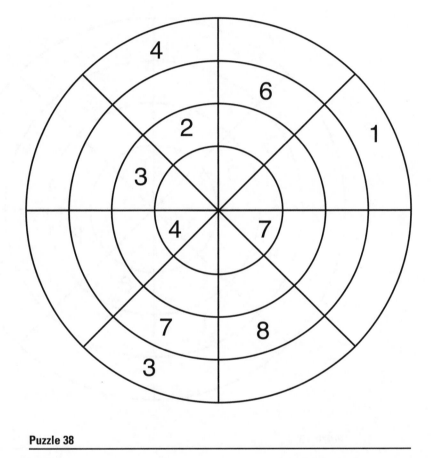

**Puzzle 38**

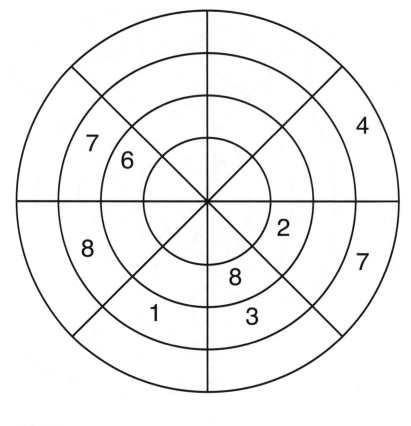

Puzzle 39

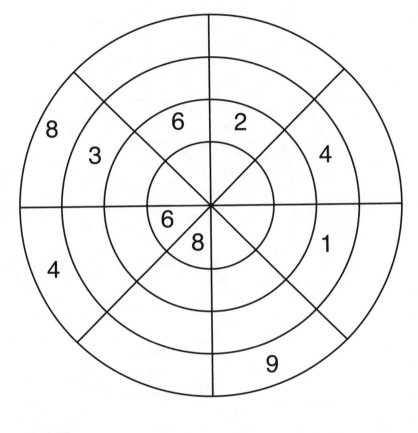

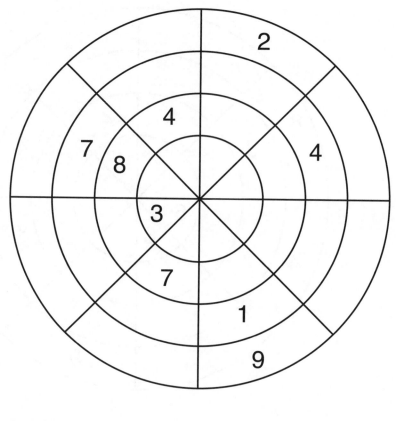

# Chapter 17

# Logic Games

● ● ● ● ● ● ● ● ● ● ● ● ● ● ● ● ● ● ● ● ● ● ● ● ● ● ● ● ● ● ● ● ● ● ● ● ● ● ● ● ● ● ● ● ●

*In This Chapter*

▶ Puzzling out logic puzzles

▶ Solving riddles

● ● ● ● ● ● ● ● ● ● ● ● ● ● ● ● ● ● ● ● ● ● ● ● ● ● ● ● ● ● ● ● ● ● ● ● ● ● ● ● ● ● ● ● ●

*I*n this chapter, I provide puzzles where you can test your logic and reasoning skills to the limit. Try your hand at logic puzzles, riddles, and cryptograms.

# Logic Puzzles

*Logic puzzles* can take a variety of forms. They may involve words, numbers, or images, and – like all puzzles – can range from being fairly easy to solve to extremely difficult.

Preparing to solve logic puzzles isn't like preparing to do a word search (see Chapter 15) or a Sudoku puzzle (see Chapter 16). You don't need to understand how the puzzle is constructed or what the rules are. You don't even have many specific strategies that you need to consider. However, you do need to be prepared to think a little more creatively, so keep the following points in mind:

✔ As with other puzzle types, each logic puzzle has a unique answer. The puzzle constructor doesn't intend for you to be able to solve one puzzle in multiple ways.

✔ In many cases, the person writing the puzzle is intention-ally veiling the answer. The way the puzzle is written may be deceptive to some degree – the degree of deception being one determinant of its level of difficulty.

Logic puzzles are a varied lot. You'll quite likely find that some answers spring to mind as soon as you've read the puzzle – your own logic will make them seem obvious to you. But others will be much more diabolical.

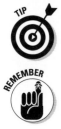

If you spend a good amount of time studying one puzzle and just can't seem to figure out the solution, walk away and come back later. A fresh look may be your best bet, or you may want to enlist help from a friend or family member.

Try to keep the answer pages closed until you've given each puzzle a good effort. You want the best workout your mind can get, and sometimes that means letting yourself get a little frustrated.

# *Easy*

### Puzzle 42

How many times can a mathematician subtract ten from 100?

### Puzzle 43

Decipher this clue: YYYMEN

# *Tricky*

### Puzzle 44

A woman gave birth to two boys on the same day, in the same year, within minutes of each other, yet the boys weren't twins. How is this possible?

### Puzzle 45

Add one line, and one line only, to make the following statement correct: 5 + 5 + 5 = 550

### Puzzle 46

Alexander is a great magician, skilled in many things. He weighs exactly 90 kilograms and is about to cross a bridge with a strict weight limit of 100 kilograms. The problem is, he's carrying three pieces of gold, each weighing 5 kilograms each. The gold puts him 5 kilograms over the strict weight limit. What can Alexander do to cross the bridge safely with all three pieces of gold?

# Tough

**Puzzle 47**

Two people stand on opposite corners of a handkerchief. They don't stretch or alter the handkerchief in any possible way. How can the people both stand on the handkerchief simultaneously without having any possibility whatsoever of touching each other?

**Puzzle 48**

Under what circumstance could a person walk along a railway track, discover an oncoming train, and have to run *towards* the train to avoid being struck?

**Puzzle 49**

Imagine this scenario. You have an extremely valuable item you need to send in the mail to an acquaintance. You have a special container that has the perfect amount of space for the item, but no extra space whatsoever. The container does, however, have a place for locks on the outside. You have locks and keys, but your acquaintance doesn't have keys to unlock any of your locks. How can you send the extremely valuable container using your lock, and have, eventually, your acquaintance be able to open the package?

# Treacherous

**Puzzle 50**

In a remote country a brutal monarch sentenced a man to death. Feeling godly, the brutal monarch told the man he'd allow one final statement. The monarch advised the man that if he lied in his final statement, he'd be drowned, but if he told the truth in his final statement, he'd be shot by firing squad. The man thought, and made his final statement. Due to the statement, the monarch was forced to release the man unharmed. What could the man possibly have said?

**Puzzle 51**

An English word that's nine letters long can form a new word each time you remove one letter. In fact, the word can change to a new word every time you remove a letter until only one letter remains. What's the word, and what's the sequence of words formed by removing one letter at a time?

# Riddles

If logic puzzles appeal to you, riddles likely will as well. These two types of puzzles are close cousins, but *riddles* are often shorter than logic puzzles and involve plays on language. For example,

> What becomes larger the more you take away from it, and smaller the more you add to it?

The answer is, *a hole in the ground.*

The reason this riddle works is because it forces you to think in a new way – to realise that not everything gets larger when you add to it.

Riddles are a great way to introduce kids to the joy of playing with language. And for adults, riddles are a great way to keep the mental gears cranking even when you've only a short time each day to devote to puzzling.

As with logic puzzles and other puzzle types, each riddle should have just one unique answer. If you can think of two or more reasonable answers to the same riddle, chances are you've outwitted the puzzle constructor!

## Easy

**Puzzle 52**

What becomes larger the more you take away from it, and smaller the more you add to it?

**Puzzle 53**

What grows up at the same time it grows down?

**Puzzle 54**

What gets larger as it eats, but smaller as it drinks?

# Tricky

**Puzzle 55**

What has a foot on either side and another foot in the middle?

**Puzzle 56**

Although it's always before you, what is it you can never see?

**Puzzle 57**

What's constantly coming but never actually arrives?

**Puzzle 58**

What goes up and down without actually moving?

# Tough

**Puzzle 59**

What's impossible to hold for more than several minutes although it's lighter than a feather?

**Puzzle 60**

Girls have it but boys don't. It's in your windows but not your walls. It's in everyone's life but not in anyone's death. What is it?

**Puzzle 61**

There are two Ws in front of two other Ws. There are two Ws behind two other Ws. There are two Ws beside two other Ws. How many Ws are there in all?

### Puzzle 62

*Homonyms* are words that are spelled differently but sound exactly the same. One pair of homonyms is unique in that although they are true homonyms, the two words are also exact opposites of each other. What are the two words?

## Treacherous

### Puzzle 63

You have a balance-type scale with two trays and seemingly nine identical coins, except that one of the coins is a fake. The weight of the fake coin is slightly less than the authentic coins. What's the easiest way to find the fake gold coin?

### Puzzle 64

What word can you read left to right or right to left, and write forwards, backwards, or upside down?

### Puzzle 65

Which two English words have three consecutive repeated letters?

### Puzzle 66

It's more powerful than God. The poorest of the poor have it. The richest of the rich need it. If you eat it or drink it, you'll die. What is it?

## Cryptograms

A *cryptogram* is a sentence or phrase that's *encrypted* or *enciphered.* What does that mean? Each letter is substituted by a different letter. (In some cases people use non-letter characters – such as numbers – as substitutions as well, but in this book I use only letters.) So within the sentence or phrase, for example, every A may be replaced with an N, and every S replaced with a P. In order to figure out what the sentence or phrase says, you have to figure out each substitution – not an easy task!

Cryptograms are more complicated than word searches and word scrambles, and they'll almost certainly require more of your time. But solving a cryptogram is really satisfying – it makes you feel like a master detective – so the extra time you spend is well worth it.

If you get stuck, make some guesses based on what you've figured out so far. And walk away if you need to – you're better off coming back to the puzzle with fresh eyes later than getting frustrated!

Here I encrypt a phrase or sentence – I substitute each letter with a different letter or character. To know what the sentence or phrase says, figure out each substitution. I give a hint for each puzzle. Keep scrap paper close by in case you need to write down your workings.

# *Easy*

**Puzzle 67**

BJVAY JSN CYP FULBN BJVAYI FOCY QUV. IBPPK JSN QUV IBPPK JBUSP.

**Hint:** The letter E appears five times.

**Puzzle 68**

UP YIGPBXW QB RQXG FNQXJNFD. FNPR ZIR UPYQZP AQGOD IF IVR ZQZPVF.

**Hint:** The letter E appears six times.

**Puzzle 69**

NOWY AJUSYSNN. AC AN COS ZWNC COLC LCCLFOSN ACNSUR CE COS GENC VZAUUALYC GSCLUN.

**Hint:** The letter H appears five times.

**Puzzle 70**

QD Q OLKG SLBG ND VZ SULBLSOGB, VZ BGIMOLOQNY XQWW OLKG SLBG ND QOPGWD.

**Hint:** The letter I appears five times.

# Tricky

**Puzzle 71**

OA GOJ AFXZKRTFOAF OTF ZVNEPAYX KB YJTFA ZYL WJPPZYL
FOJGF XOZX OTF VAZFJY TF GAZS

**Hint:** The letter H appears seven times.

**Puzzle 72**

QCHPHKHN B ZHHV VBFH HMHNUBTBPY, B VBH RXQP OPWBV
WCH ZHHVBPY LGTTHT.

**Hint:** The letter B isn't used at all.

**Puzzle 73**

FEIDF UVIE VSC JCDFJCAF. UVIE BJDFPXND BJKHF PD SNWW ON
UVIE VSC JCDFNPR VG DVBNVCN NWDN'D.

**Hint:** The letter H appears just once.

**Puzzle 74**

WAG MIER CGMCEG OAM ELTWGI WM QMWA TLHGT MP S
PSKLER ZVSXXGE SXG WAG IGFW HMMX IGLJAQMVXT.

**Hint:** The letter X appears just once.

**Puzzle 75**

GSS LBO DOGTLYKTS HOALYUOALH YA LBO ZNFSX ZOYJB SOHH
LBGA G HYAJSO SNPOSM GWLYNA.

**Hint:** The letter I appears six times.

**Puzzle 76**

VKMDM'Q SEVKYSF YS VKM HYTTGM EZ VKM DEPT ORV
XMGGEA QVDYUMQ PST TMPT PDHPTYGGEQ.

**Hint:** The letter I appears five times.

**Puzzle 77**

VZO ROW YFKKXV LO MXGEAZOI UEVZXBV SCEYVEXK, KXC WFK
MOCSOYVOI UEVZXBV VCEFGA.

**Hint:** THE appears only once.

# *Tough*

**Puzzle 78**

IYUYUSYI, XWYL MWY DYRJTJV ZMIAMZ WEZ ZMAQQ WY ZWTXZ
WEZ SRJVZECY MT WRGQ MWY XTIGC.

**Hint:** One word ends with O.

**Puzzle 79**

XHWZ QM KFXX CQKIG HUS SGFBI WHJOI RQGI MHFXJGIO DAHU
XHWZ QM FUDIXXFLIUWI HUS HVFXFDT.

**Hint:** The letter F appears three times.

**Puzzle 80**

QWHYWBW YI VD KVI, VKPW MZVK U IYEW, UHH EWEQWDN VT
IFW TUEYHX FUL QDWUJTUNI IVAWIFWD.

**Hint:** THE appears just once.

**Puzzle 81**

CQ HLI XCPP MYTRN ULVT FCUT MDSVYTRCRB FDT SJT, HLI'PP
MYTRN PTMM FCUT ZDLYYCRB XLLN.

**Hint:** The letter G appears twice.

**Puzzle 82**

ZQA NXYOQTL DXOZ PKKALZPIUA ZX MXC KXDAO EYXD P
ZQPVFESU PVC KQAAYESU QAPYZ.

**Hint:** The letters EE appear once.

**Puzzle 83**

_____

ZNO GHRF PV UBGL HRF NPROX NHD BZD FKHTSHJLD. XPA JHR
QOZ LBJLOF SX H JPT HRF DZARQ SX H SOO.

**Hint:** The letter K appears four times.

**Puzzle 84**

_____

YDGF L ZLF RGGR ODG DLFSYXQOQFE CF ODG YLNN, ODGXG QR
MXCKLKNP L TDQNS QF ODG HLZQNP.

**Hint:** The letter U isn't used at all.

# *Treacherous*

**Puzzle 85**

_____

LSOQJDCIZFG PCD JLSD YJJOQ MXF JDIG PACOCPFSO PCD NSSL
FASE JLSD.

**Hint:** The letter K appears just once.

**Puzzle 86**

_____

NRL'W QRZRGGRS SDCC IV IVQQVG QXEU EUH HVWQVGLEH HRO
XEBV VBVG PURSU.

**Hint:** The letter C isn't used at all.

**Puzzle 87**

_____

JSNI HLTEXV QS ESH ASUG MYAW; HLG VDSWGE RSIQ, HLG VLSH
YIISR, HLG DYVH PTJG YEQ HLG EGXPGAHGQ SDDSIHNETHZ.

**Hint:** The letter W appears twice.

**Puzzle 88**

_____

C ZCQDNNF BQJV VUDA ECXACQHICXURX SDQ ZOJS AUR
GRDXAX: ZCQDQYCDN VJOOCRX.

**Hint:** The letter P isn't used at all.

**Puzzle 89**

YD AGTTJDY TD HNNHEZCGMMS QDUT ZXH RJYK DN GMM JZT ADBHQT DN GEZJYV GYK QHGTDYJYV GT NHGQ.

**Hint:** The letter B appears just once.

**Puzzle 90**

ZNKQYNM OG UPY FKRKFOUM US RYNHSNC RNSRYNAM YQYD BPYD GFKNYT PKAH US TYKUP.

**Hint:** The letter W appears just once.

**Puzzle 91**

NHHNLBEQZBJ ZC OZCCAG WJ ONCB HANHMA WATXECA ZB ZC GLACCAG ZQ NIALXMMC XQG MNNVC MZVA PNLV.

**Hint:** The letter H isn't used at all.

# Part VI
# The Part of Tens

The 5<sup>th</sup> Wave

By Rich Tennant

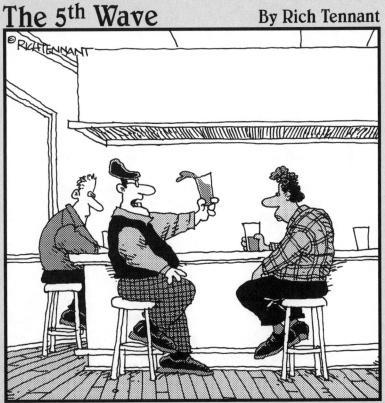

"My wife wants me to improve my brain by switching hands when performing regular tasks, but darn if it isn't awkward holding a pint up with my left hand."

# *In this part...*

*I*n this part you find great tips on brain training, along with ten exciting, new things that you can try to expand your brain. And you can also train your brain on the move – find out ten top tips for scientifically proven activities that make your brain work better.

# Chapter 18

# Ten New Habits to Train Your Brain

*Y*ou can easily get stuck in a rut – waking up and doing the same thing day in and day out. Well, today is the day to make a change. The idea that learning something new is a great way to keep your brain sharp has a scientific basis. Each day your hippocampus sees new neurons generated to help with learning and memory (for information on the hippocampus, see Chapter 2). When you learn something new, you keep these neurons active and can slow down cognitive decline. In this chapter I give you ten ideas you can choose from to make a start in training your brain to keep it healthy and sharp.

## Try Line Dancing

If you think that line dancing is reserved for dusty bars filled with smoke swirls and cowboy boots, think again. Line dancing not only keeps your body fit, but it also increases serotonin levels, which makes your brain feel good. *Line dancing*, as the name suggests, is where you stand in a line and follow a sequence of steps around the room. Line dancing isn't as easy as it looks, but it certainly is fun.

And you can choose from many different routines and steps. When you're learning new steps, you're challenging your brain to stay active. So grab a partner by the hand and head to the nearest saloon! Cowboy boots optional.

Here are some dancing tips to get you going:

✔ **Don't look at your feet.** Line dancing works better if you look up at the teacher, or your DVD. Try to see yourself doing the dance steps in your head and resist the urge to keep looking down, or even at the person's feet in front of you. When you look up, you can take in information on how your body and feet should be moving. When you look down, it's easy to get distracted and feel discouraged if your feet aren't doing what you want. So, eyes up and feet moving!

✔ **Memorise the steps.** Committing the steps to memory is a great way to train your brain. You're encouraging your brain to learn something new and commit it to long-term memory. You can also enjoy the experience much more if you don't have to keep worrying about what comes next in the dance routine.

✔ **Think ahead.** Anticipate the next step in the routine. Close your eyes and think of what your feet should be doing next. This way, you're training your brain to keep a set of dance sequences in your memory rather than simply following what everyone else is doing. By anticipating the next move, you're using your spatial skills (see Chapter 7).

Don't give up on this idea if you can't find a class in your area or a teacher that you like. Going to a *ceilidh* (an evening of traditional music and dancing) is a great alternative. Although you can't wear your cowboy boots, a ceilidh is just as much fun as line dancing, and it also boosts your brain power.

Another option is to invest in a DVD about dancing. There are so many to choose from, and when you buy from a site like Amazon you also have the benefit of reading reviews from other buyers to help you make your choice.

## Puzzle Over Jigsaws

Jigsaw puzzles aren't just for kids. Doing a jigsaw is a great way to boost co-ordination and spatial thinking.

If you feel that you haven't done puzzles in a while and can't start, just choose something easy to start off with. Don't attempt a 1,000-piece puzzle of scenery! Start with a jigsaw of a picture that you love, maybe a favourite animal or a familiar painting. This way, you can draw on your knowledge of the image in your head to complete the puzzle.

Before you begin your jigsaw, be sure to follow these steps:

1. **Face up.** Before you start your puzzle, the first thing to do is to make sure that all the pieces are facing upwards. This may be time consuming, but it's worth doing because your puzzle time goes a lot more smoothly and is more enjoyable as a result. And if you're having a good time then you're more likely to keep doing jigsaws! While you're turning the pieces face up, you can also sort them into piles by colour or create a separate pile for the corner and border pieces of the puzzle.

2. **Head to the border.** The next step is to put the border together. This is relatively easy but makes your 'puzzling' a lot easier. If you can't find some of the border pieces, don't spend too long looking. Just keep the space empty and they'll turn up along the way.

3. **Section off.** Next, start tackling your piles. Start with the easiest ones first. Some people find it best to start with large objects in the puzzles because they have variety and as a result they're easier to put together. Others find sorting according to colour is a great way to begin.

The key is to avoid getting frustrated and remember: start with an easy puzzle. You don't want to give yourself such a hard challenge that you never even finish your first puzzle.

# *Learn a Language*

With so many budget airlines, going on a quick weekend getaway has never been easier. And what better excuse to learn a language than to be able to order an Italian gelato on a hot day, or to bargain for that must-have item in a market place in an exotic location?

But other than the satisfaction of feeling like a local while on holiday, learning a language also has tremendous benefits for your brain. Brain scans show that people who are bilingual have denser grey matter in the part of the brain linked to visual-spatial skills (the parietal cortex, see Chapter 2).

With so many digital resources, learning a language has become even easier. From the *For Dummies* series with its wide selection of different language titles to suit your interest (along with language learning i-phone apps) to free online sound clips of common phrases, you've no reason not to spend even ten minutes each day learning new words and phrases.

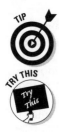

Knowing you'll have an opportunity to use your new skill helps. So try to learn the language of a place you're planning to visit in the near future.

If you're planning a 'stay-cation' instead, then here are some suggestions for how to practise your language skills at home:

- **Find a friend.** Strike up a friendship with a fellow language learner or even a native speaker. Then make a plan to meet up and only speak in that language. You may find the conversation tricky at first, but you'll find yourself learning the language much more quickly. Pick a venue, like a café or a restaurant, so that you can practise phrases to use before you meet.

- **Read a book.** Most local libraries have language books that come with a CD. If you don't want to invest in a language programme then the local library is the stop for you. A great way to practise your language is to seek out children's books written in the language you're learning; check out popular children's books, ranging from very simple ones (with a single word on a page) to books with more complex stories, at your library. Often libraries have story books with English and another language on the same page so you can learn new words as well as feel like a child again!

- **Sing a song.** Songs are a fun and catchy way to remember new phrases. The rhythm, the lyrics – learning something new is easier when you're just humming along. So turn up the volume. Who knows, you may even learn a phrase or two to make your holiday more romantic!

# Memorise Capital Cities

I remember pouring over a world map as child, staring at the shapes of the countries, thinking about what it would be like to live there, what animals there were, what kind of food they have. But most of all, I remember playing games with my brother to 'guess the capitals'. My mother would list a country, and we'd try to guess the capital. It was a fun way for us to discover a little bit more about a different place. Little did we know that we were also training our memory along the way! Flip back to Chapters 4 and 5 to find out more about improving your memory.

Events like the World Cup and the Olympics give you many opportunities to find out about world capitals and their flags.

If memorising capitals reminds you of school days, it shouldn't. Make this activity fun! My little boy loved matching all the flags with the football teams that were part of the World Cup. He didn't even realise that he was learning something along the way. Now he loves picking out the different flags whenever I show them to him.

You can make this activity fun for yourself as well. Have a race with a friend and see how many capitals and countries you can name – loser buys dinner! Or race against the clock: set the timer for 60 seconds and list as many capitals as you can remember. You can play with flags as well, or even list one fact about a country. Just remember to enjoy yourself.

# Walk in a Different Park

A change of scene can make a big difference to your mental health. You don't need to make a drastic change – like moving to a new city. But small changes can make a huge difference. For example, if you take the dog for a walk in the same place every day, change your route today!

You may not realise this but looking at the same trees or flowers each day may be dragging you down. Finding somewhere new to go for a walk is a quick pick up. You may be surprised at how energised you feel by getting the opportunity to look at new surroundings. Think of how refreshed you feel when you return from a holiday – your eyes are sparkling, your worries have rolled away, and you feel that all is right and wonderful in the world. You can recreate the experience to a small degree when you change your physical surroundings.

If you usually walk or cycle to work, change your route every so often. If you can leave work earlier one day, take a longer and more scenic way home. Stop to enjoy the birds singing and the flowers blooming. Think of one beautiful thing that you see on your journey.

# Eat New Food

In Chapter 12 I talk about food that you can eat to make your brain smart. Try to eat something new from that list. If you've never eaten salmon, try some today.

Sharing experiences with a friend is always more fun. So if you can't pluck up the courage to try a new food on your own, invite a friend along. Encourage your friend to try something new as well.

That way you can both get the benefits of brain-boosting foods and enjoy each other's company.

Your whole menu doesn't have to consist of new food. Just add one item to begin with. It's great if you can try to eat a new food once a month.

# Join a Book Club

A book club is a great way to flex your mental muscles. Although reading is a great activity, discussing what you read with a group of friends is even better. A book club is a fantastic way to share ideas and discover new things as well.

If there isn't a book club near you, start one yourself. Here are some tips to get you going:

- **Find a time.** The first thing to do is to pick a time that's best suited for you and your friends. For example, if you have to drop children off at school, meet up after that. Or if you're rushing off to work, then maybe an evening would work best. The important thing is to make your book club part of your schedule to relax, rather than viewing it as a chore or an extra activity that you have to do.

- **Don't forget the nibbles.** Everything seems better with snacks! If you're hosting the book club, you don't have to slave for hours in the kitchen. Something simple, such as vegetables and dips, is fine, or you can rotate so that each person takes turns to bring something along. This takes the pressure off you, but also makes sure that everyone has something to munch on while you discuss a book.

- **Choose your books.** Of course, the most important part of the book club is the book! Pick a different genre for each month. You can start with a detective novel for one month and then switch to a different genre the following month – maybe a popular science book.

  You can also pick fiction best sellers to start off with. Often best sellers are made into films, so you can have some idea of the plot before you start reading.

  Don't feel that you have to read the whole book each time. Some book clubs just read a few chapters to discuss.

Circulating a list of talking points to get the conversation going can be helpful. Talking points can be as simple as 'What did you like about the book?' to discussing a character's motivations for her actions. You can also extend the discussion to include how you'd act if you were in a character's situation. If the book has been made into a movie, you can compare strengths and weaknesses of the two story lines. The whole point is to create an opportunity to exchange ideas about a topic that interests you.

# Write a Film Review

Everyone's a critic! And so you should be too. Writing regularly can help you to preserve your cognitive skills, so try starting with a film review. Think of one thing that you liked and another thing that you didn't like about the film and write about 100 words explaining your views. Make yourself think carefully about why you've chosen certain aspects of the film to focus on. Honing in on one or two ideas is better, because then it becomes more manageable to talk about the film.

Here are some tips to get you started on becoming the next Barry Norman or Roger Ebert:

✔ **Save the yelling.** Training yourself to be logical in a review is more beneficial to you than being emotional, so try to avoid ranting in your review. Instead, form your arguments for your review in a careful and considered way. If you can, don't make generalisations about your views. Be as specific as you can in your arguments. Think of one scene to focus on and use that as an example of what you liked or didn't like about the movie.

✔ **Become a budding movie buff.** It may help to compare the movie to another movie to illustrate how it was better or worse. Having an 'anchor' can help develop your ideas. Comparing two things helps your brain make connections between different ideas. You may find that you become better in everyday conversations as a result!

✔ **Publish it!** If you feel brave enough, you can even publish your review. Many websites like Rotten Tomatoes (www.rotten tomatoes.com) lets readers leave their own comments and reviews on a movie, and some online newspaper forums do as well. If you're really serious about taking this further and view yourself as a budding critic, try this site: www.everyonesa critic.net.

# Spend Five Minutes Each Morning in Contemplation

Your mental health is crucial to how your brain functioning works (see Chapter 9). So don't let your problems overwhelm you. Spend each morning preparing for the day by finding a few moments of calm and contemplation.

You may need to wake up a little earlier so you can escape the morning madness in your house. But it's worth doing so. I always find that my day goes a lot better when I've had a few moments in the morning to myself before everyone else wakes up. It may be that you just have a cup of coffee or tea and mentally prepare for the day. Or maybe you just like to sit and enjoy the silence.

Spend your quiet moments however you choose, but just don't pass on this one – it can set your mind right for the day. (Check out *Mindfulness For Dummies* by Shamash Alidina for more tips and advice.)

# List Three Things You're Thankful for Before Bed

A happy heart makes a healthy brain. Sometimes feeling frazzled at the end of the day is easy. Between work responsibilities, family commitments, and a whole host of other obligations, you may even find it hard to fall asleep at night because your mind won't stop buzzing.

Put all those thoughts aside and focus on three things that happened that day that you're thankful for. It may be a simple thing, like your morning coffee, or a smile from your child, or a surprise phone call from a loved one. Focus on each of these moments and say out aloud what they are and why they made you happy. Hearing yourself say these happy thoughts before bed is sure to put a smile on your face and give you sweet dreams. After all, you have tomorrow to figure out solutions to everything else.

# Chapter 19

# Ten Brain Games to Play on the Move

### In This Chapter

▶ Training your brain anywhere

▶ Findings ways to boost your brain as you move

on't let the lack of time be a reason for you not to train your brain. This chapter lists ten games that you can play on the move. So if you're busy commuting or travelling, use that time to play some of these games. Just make sure that you're not driving at the time!

## Match That Face

The next time you're flipping through the newspaper or a magazine and spot a face you recognise, list three things that you remember about the person. The person may be a politician, an actor, or a singer. Whoever he is, try to think hard to come up with facts that you know about the person.

You can also do this with friends. Look through a yearbook from school or an old photo album. You may recognise the face but not the name. This is a great opportunity to get your brain working to remember not only someone's name, but also a fact about him. It may be something like – 'I sat next to him in chemistry class', or 'We used to exchange jokes during music class'. The key is to keep your brain active by practising these links and not letting them grow weak. Read Chapter 7 for more tips on this topic.

## Spot the Objects

This game is great for when you go to a new place. If you're waiting at a doctor's office or in a café, why not try this game? Look around the room for one minute – time yourself. Now close your eyes and think of ten things that you saw in the room. Give yourself ten seconds to come up with these objects. Describe them in as much detail as you can remember. For example, if you remember a magazine on the table, don't just say *magazine*. Think of the title of the magazine, what was on the cover, any key words that stood out? What about a plant? Did you see one in the room? Think of as much detail as possible.

Would you like to make it more of a challenge? Try this. Give yourself only ten seconds to remember 20 things in the room. Here also, don't just name the objects, but try to also remember features about them.

Resist the urge to peek – you want to train your visual memory to pick up on cues around you as fast as possible. Read Chapter 7 for more information on boosting your visual and spatial memory skills to improve your ability to remember faces and directions.

# Tip-of-the-tongue Game

Pick a category. Let's say *food*. Now set a time limit – how about one minute? Name as many foods as you can in one minute. How did you do? Most people can name around 30 food items. Push yourself to beat this number. Go for 60 items.

Here's another way you can make it harder. Pick a category and a time limit. Now pick a letter – say the letter *D*. Now name as many foods as you can that start with the letter D in 30 seconds.

You can have word 'races' with your friends to see who can name more food. Don't forget to keep your eye on the timer. A key part of this training game is to come up with as many items as you can in a short space of time. This trains your brain to think faster.

# Number Game

Start with a high number like 100 and then count backwards in twos. So you'd count 100, 98, 96, 94 and so on. That was an easy one.

Make it harder by counting backwards in threes or fours. And if you really want to give yourself a challenge, give yourself a time limit. Or if you want to make it even harder, then do something else while you're counting backwards, like tapping your foot.

Sometimes doing two things at the same time can get confusing. By training your brain this way, you get better at managing doing multiple things at the same time. This is a great game to play while brushing your teeth or doing something that doesn't really require you to do much thinking.

# Memory Game

This game is called the *n-back* task, where you have to remember something back in a sequence that you saw. Psychologists found that people who trained using these types of activities three times a week for 20 weeks improved their IQ and memory scores.

Here's what you do. Get a friend to read out the letters that follow. Every time he sees a letter shown in **bold**, he asks you to decide whether you heard that same letter three letters back.

X C E B **S** E I X O **S** X P O W E Q **W** X K H K (and so on)

For example, for the letter *E*, the answer is yes; for the letter *S*, the answer is no. You can also do this activity with shapes or pictures.

Too easy? Try doing the same activity but now do it while singing your favourite song.

Still too easy? Try doing the same activity, but decide whether you saw the same letter (or shape or picture) three letters (or shapes or pictures) back *and* sing your favourite song.

Can't get a friend to help out? Try this game with cars on the road. Just remember the colour of the car. Then every so often ask yourself whether you saw a red car two cars back, and so on. It's harder than it sounds!

# Tell Me a Story

This is a great game to do when you're bored and waiting at a train station or an airport. Find someone who looks interesting. Now come up with a story for the person. Why is he there? Is he leaving or arriving? What's the reason for his trip?

The goal of this activity is to get your creative juice going. Imagine that you're a novelist and the person is a character in your story. Create motivations for him, reasons for his actions. Think of what would happen next in your story. Be as creative as you want; after all, this is your story. Read Chapter 8 on the benefits of a creative brain.

# Drumming for your Brain

You need a friend to help you with this one, but it's a great activity to do while you're waiting. Ask your friend to hum a tune in his head. But he can't tell you what the song is. Next, ask him to tap the tune's rhythm out on the table.

Listen carefully, and then tap the rhythm out as soon as your friend's finished. See if you can remember the rhythm. Try to get as much of the beat correct. Your memory for rhythm is closely connected to your memory for language. By training how well you can remember a particular rhythm, you're boosting your language skills as well. Read Chapter 8 for the benefits of music for the brain.

# Read a Challenging Book

Don't just be content with reading your usual newspaper or magazine. Why not challenge yourself by picking up something new to read? If you usually read fiction, pick up a historical novel instead. Reading something new is a great way to expand your horizons and get your brain thinking in new ways. If you're not sure what to pick, online bookstores like Amazon rank the bestselling books, as well as providing customer reviews. So you can read what other people think before you dive in. For some books, you can even read a section or two inside before you buy. Whatever you end up choosing, the important thing is that you try new reading material.

# Circling Fun

If you really can't part with your daily paper, then here's an activity that you can do with your newspaper or magazine. Grab a pen and set your watch for this activity. Follow these steps:

1. **Decide on a time limit.**

   Start with ten seconds.

2. **Pick a word.**

   Let's say the word *then*.

3. **Grab your pen and circle as many *then*s as you see on the page in ten seconds.**

This game is great for training your visual skills and for learning to spot visual cues quickly, and training your brain for speed.

# *Wrapping It Up. . .*

I can't end this chapter without encouraging you to do the fantastic brain games that I provide in Chapters 15, 16 and 17. Take your pick from easy, tough, or treacherous options in crosswords, word puzzles, logic games, and Sudoku. The chapters have something for everyone and are guaranteed to get your brain working.

If you're looking for more of challenge after you've completed the brain games in those chapters, why not turn to *Brain Games For Dummies* by Timothy E. Parker for more games to help keep your brain working well.

# Appendix

# The Payoff: Checking Your Answers

• • • • • • • • • • • • • • • • • • • • • • • • • • • • • • • • • • • •

*P*lease don't read through this appendix until you've worked on the puzzles in Chapters 15 to 17!

**Puzzle 1**

LIVES

**Puzzle 2**

CO-STAR

**Puzzle 3**

SORES

**Puzzle 4**

SECURE

**Puzzle 5**

LISTEN

**Puzzle 6**

THEY SEE

**Puzzle 7**

THEIRS

**Puzzle 8**

SOBER

**Puzzle 9**

SPEND IT

**Puzzle 10**

CHEATING

**Puzzle 11**

KITCHEN

**Puzzle 12**

DEBIT CARD

**Puzzle 13**

DATE'S UP

**Puzzle 14**

THE CLASSROOM

**Puzzle 15**

CAR INSURANCE

**Puzzle 16**

DETECT THIEVES

**Puzzle 17**

ELEVEN PLUS TWO

**Puzzle 18**

THE DESERT REGION

**Puzzle 19**

PAID ME EVERY CENT

**Puzzle 20**

CASH LOST IN 'EM

**Puzzle 21**

DREAM FOR CUE BALLS

**Puzzle 22**

NEW YEAR'S RESOLUTION

**Puzzle 23**

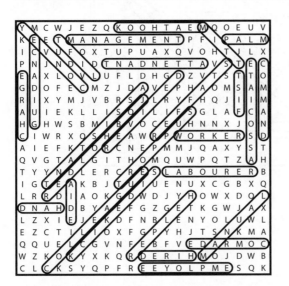

### Puzzle 24

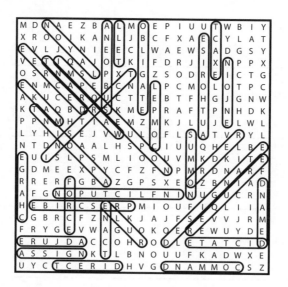

### Puzzle 25

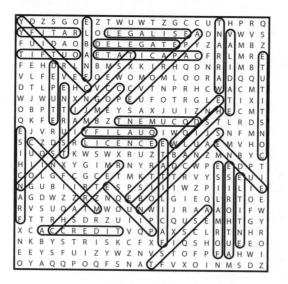

**Puzzle 26**

| 1 | 2 | 4 | 7 | 3 | 6 | 8 | 9 | 5 |
|---|---|---|---|---|---|---|---|---|
| 3 | 5 | 8 | 9 | 1 | 4 | 6 | 7 | 2 |
| 6 | 9 | 7 | 8 | 5 | 2 | 4 | 1 | 3 |
| 8 | 3 | 1 | 6 | 4 | 5 | 7 | 2 | 9 |
| 9 | 4 | 5 | 2 | 7 | 1 | 3 | 8 | 6 |
| 2 | 7 | 6 | 3 | 8 | 9 | 5 | 4 | 1 |
| 7 | 8 | 9 | 1 | 6 | 3 | 2 | 5 | 4 |
| 5 | 1 | 3 | 4 | 2 | 7 | 9 | 6 | 8 |
| 4 | 6 | 2 | 5 | 9 | 8 | 1 | 3 | 7 |

**Puzzle 27**

| 2 | 5 | 4 | 6 | 3 | 9 | 1 | 7 | 8 |
|---|---|---|---|---|---|---|---|---|
| 9 | 8 | 6 | 7 | 4 | 1 | 5 | 3 | 2 |
| 1 | 3 | 7 | 8 | 2 | 5 | 4 | 9 | 6 |
| 6 | 1 | 5 | 3 | 9 | 4 | 8 | 2 | 7 |
| 7 | 9 | 2 | 1 | 5 | 8 | 6 | 4 | 3 |
| 3 | 4 | 8 | 2 | 6 | 7 | 9 | 1 | 5 |
| 8 | 6 | 1 | 9 | 7 | 2 | 3 | 5 | 4 |
| 5 | 7 | 3 | 4 | 1 | 6 | 2 | 8 | 9 |
| 4 | 2 | 9 | 5 | 8 | 3 | 7 | 6 | 1 |

**Puzzle 28**

| 3 | 7 | 1 | 8 | 5 | 6 | 9 | 2 | 4 |
|---|---|---|---|---|---|---|---|---|
| 4 | 9 | 5 | 2 | 1 | 7 | 3 | 6 | 8 |
| 6 | 2 | 8 | 4 | 3 | 9 | 1 | 5 | 7 |
| 9 | 4 | 6 | 7 | 2 | 1 | 5 | 8 | 3 |
| 5 | 8 | 7 | 6 | 4 | 3 | 2 | 1 | 9 |
| 1 | 3 | 2 | 5 | 9 | 8 | 4 | 7 | 6 |
| 7 | 5 | 9 | 1 | 8 | 4 | 6 | 3 | 2 |
| 2 | 6 | 3 | 9 | 7 | 5 | 8 | 4 | 1 |
| 8 | 1 | 4 | 3 | 6 | 2 | 7 | 9 | 5 |

### Puzzle 29

| 9 | 7 | 5 | 8 | 2 | 1 | 3 | 4 | 6 |
|---|---|---|---|---|---|---|---|---|
| 6 | 3 | 2 | 4 | 5 | 7 | 1 | 8 | 9 |
| 4 | 1 | 8 | 3 | 6 | 9 | 5 | 7 | 2 |
| 2 | 6 | 1 | 5 | 4 | 3 | 8 | 9 | 7 |
| 8 | 5 | 4 | 9 | 7 | 2 | 6 | 3 | 1 |
| 7 | 9 | 3 | 1 | 8 | 6 | 4 | 2 | 5 |
| 3 | 4 | 9 | 7 | 1 | 5 | 2 | 6 | 8 |
| 1 | 2 | 7 | 6 | 3 | 8 | 9 | 5 | 4 |
| 5 | 8 | 6 | 2 | 9 | 4 | 7 | 1 | 3 |

### Puzzle 30

| 8 | 5 | 9 | 7 | 1 | 2 | 3 | 6 | 4 |
|---|---|---|---|---|---|---|---|---|
| 7 | 3 | 2 | 5 | 4 | 6 | 8 | 9 | 1 |
| 1 | 6 | 4 | 9 | 8 | 3 | 2 | 7 | 5 |
| 3 | 7 | 1 | 8 | 9 | 5 | 6 | 4 | 2 |
| 4 | 2 | 6 | 1 | 3 | 7 | 5 | 8 | 9 |
| 9 | 8 | 5 | 2 | 6 | 4 | 1 | 3 | 7 |
| 2 | 9 | 3 | 6 | 7 | 1 | 4 | 5 | 8 |
| 5 | 4 | 8 | 3 | 2 | 9 | 7 | 1 | 6 |
| 6 | 1 | 7 | 4 | 5 | 8 | 9 | 2 | 3 |

### Puzzle 31

| 6 | 7 | 8 | 4 | 5 | 2 | 1 | 3 | 9 |
|---|---|---|---|---|---|---|---|---|
| 9 | 5 | 2 | 8 | 3 | 1 | 7 | 6 | 4 |
| 4 | 3 | 1 | 7 | 9 | 6 | 5 | 8 | 2 |
| 3 | 2 | 4 | 6 | 1 | 9 | 8 | 7 | 5 |
| 5 | 8 | 6 | 2 | 7 | 4 | 9 | 1 | 3 |
| 7 | 1 | 9 | 3 | 8 | 5 | 4 | 2 | 6 |
| 1 | 6 | 5 | 9 | 2 | 8 | 3 | 4 | 7 |
| 2 | 9 | 7 | 1 | 4 | 3 | 6 | 5 | 8 |
| 8 | 4 | 3 | 5 | 6 | 7 | 2 | 9 | 1 |

**Puzzle 32**

| 4 | 3 | 1 | 9 | 6 | 2 | 5 | 7 | 8 |
|---|---|---|---|---|---|---|---|---|
| 2 | 5 | 7 | 3 | 8 | 4 | 1 | 9 | 6 |
| 6 | 8 | 9 | 1 | 7 | 5 | 4 | 3 | 2 |
| 7 | 2 | 4 | 5 | 9 | 3 | 8 | 6 | 1 |
| 3 | 6 | 8 | 7 | 4 | 1 | 9 | 2 | 5 |
| 1 | 9 | 5 | 8 | 2 | 6 | 7 | 4 | 3 |
| 9 | 4 | 3 | 2 | 5 | 8 | 6 | 1 | 7 |
| 8 | 1 | 6 | 4 | 3 | 7 | 2 | 5 | 9 |
| 5 | 7 | 2 | 6 | 1 | 9 | 3 | 8 | 4 |

**Puzzle 33**

| 2 | 7 | 6 | 3 | 5 | 9 | 1 | 8 | 4 |
|---|---|---|---|---|---|---|---|---|
| 5 | 3 | 4 | 2 | 8 | 1 | 7 | 9 | 6 |
| 9 | 8 | 1 | 4 | 6 | 7 | 2 | 3 | 5 |
| 8 | 9 | 3 | 5 | 2 | 6 | 4 | 1 | 7 |
| 4 | 1 | 5 | 9 | 7 | 8 | 6 | 2 | 3 |
| 6 | 2 | 7 | 1 | 4 | 3 | 9 | 5 | 8 |
| 7 | 6 | 9 | 8 | 3 | 2 | 5 | 4 | 1 |
| 3 | 4 | 2 | 7 | 1 | 5 | 8 | 6 | 9 |
| 1 | 5 | 8 | 6 | 9 | 4 | 3 | 7 | 2 |

**Puzzle 34**

| 3 | 5 | 4 | 6 | 2 | 7 | 1 | 9 | 8 |
|---|---|---|---|---|---|---|---|---|
| 1 | 6 | 8 | 9 | 4 | 3 | 5 | 2 | 7 |
| 2 | 7 | 9 | 1 | 5 | 8 | 3 | 6 | 4 |
| 9 | 4 | 6 | 8 | 1 | 2 | 7 | 3 | 5 |
| 5 | 2 | 3 | 4 | 7 | 9 | 8 | 1 | 6 |
| 7 | 8 | 1 | 3 | 6 | 5 | 9 | 4 | 2 |
| 8 | 9 | 5 | 2 | 3 | 6 | 4 | 7 | 1 |
| 4 | 3 | 2 | 7 | 8 | 1 | 6 | 5 | 9 |
| 6 | 1 | 7 | 5 | 9 | 4 | 2 | 8 | 3 |

**Puzzle 35**

| 7 | 8 | 9 | 3 | 6 | 2 | 4 | 1 | 5 |
| 1 | 3 | 2 | 4 | 5 | 7 | 6 | 8 | 9 |
| 5 | 6 | 4 | 1 | 9 | 8 | 3 | 7 | 2 |
| 9 | 5 | 6 | 2 | 3 | 1 | 8 | 4 | 7 |
| 4 | 7 | 3 | 5 | 8 | 6 | 9 | 2 | 1 |
| 8 | 2 | 1 | 9 | 7 | 4 | 5 | 3 | 6 |
| 3 | 9 | 7 | 8 | 1 | 5 | 2 | 6 | 4 |
| 6 | 4 | 8 | 7 | 2 | 9 | 1 | 5 | 3 |
| 2 | 1 | 5 | 6 | 4 | 3 | 7 | 9 | 8 |

**Puzzle 36**

| 6 | 8 | 1 | 3 | 5 | 9 | 7 | 2 | 4 |
| 7 | 4 | 2 | 8 | 6 | 1 | 3 | 5 | 9 |
| 3 | 9 | 5 | 7 | 2 | 4 | 1 | 8 | 6 |
| 9 | 6 | 4 | 1 | 8 | 3 | 5 | 7 | 2 |
| 1 | 2 | 7 | 5 | 4 | 6 | 8 | 9 | 3 |
| 5 | 3 | 8 | 2 | 9 | 7 | 4 | 6 | 1 |
| 8 | 5 | 3 | 9 | 1 | 2 | 6 | 4 | 7 |
| 2 | 1 | 6 | 4 | 7 | 5 | 9 | 3 | 8 |
| 4 | 7 | 9 | 6 | 3 | 8 | 2 | 1 | 5 |

**Puzzle 37**

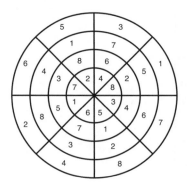

**Puzzle 38**

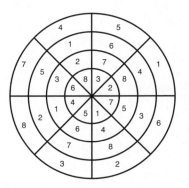

**Puzzle 39**

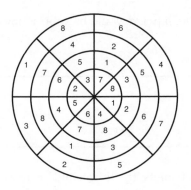

**Puzzle 40**

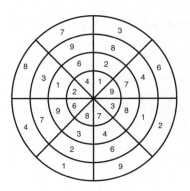

**Puzzle 41**

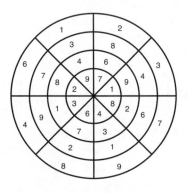

**Puzzle 42**

Once. After that, the mathematician would be subtracting 10 from 90, then 80, then 70 . . .

**Puzzle 43**

Three wise men

**Puzzle 44**

They were part of a set of triplets, the third child being a daughter.

**Puzzle 45**

5 + 5 4 5 = 550 (add one diagonal line to the second '+' to make it a '4')

**Puzzle 46**

Alexander juggles the gold as he crosses the bridge, keeping at least one piece in the air at all times.

**Puzzle 47**

One person stands on one corner of the handkerchief and closes a door. The second person stands on the corner of the handkerchief protruding under the door. With the door between them, the two people can't possibly touch.

**Puzzle 48**

The person is on tracks in a railroad tunnel walking toward the train and is close to the end when he notices the oncoming train. The person must then run forward to clear the tunnel before the train enters.

**Puzzle 49**

You send the container with one of your locks securing the container. Your acquaintance receives the container, and without trying to open it, attaches his lock next to your lock. He then sends the container back to you. You use your key to unlock your lock, remove it, and send the container back to your acquaintance with only his lock on the container. He can then open the container using his own key to his own lock.

**Puzzle 50**

The man said, 'I will be drowned.'

**Puzzle 51**

The word is startling and the word sequence is starting, staring, string, sting, sing, sin, in, I

**Puzzle 52**

A hole in the ground

**Puzzle 53**

A goose

**Puzzle 54**

A fire

**Puzzle 55**

A yardstick

**Puzzle 56**

The future

**Puzzle 57**

Tomorrow

**Puzzle 58**

Stairs

**Puzzle 59**

Your breath

**Puzzle 60**

The letter I

**Puzzle 61**

Four, positioned like this: WW WW

**Puzzle 62**

Raise and raze

**Puzzle 63**

Taking any eight of the nine coins, load the scale with four coins on either side. Whenever two sides are equal, the remaining coin is the fake.

**Puzzle 64**

NOON

**Puzzle 65**

Bookkeeper (oo-kk-ee) and sweet-toothed (ee-tt-oo)

**Puzzle 66**

Nothing

**Puzzle 67**

LAUGH AND THE WORLD LAUGHS WITH YOU. SNORE AND YOU SLEEP ALONE.

**Puzzle 68**

BE CAREFUL OF YOUR THOUGHTS. THEY MAY BECOME WORDS AT ANY MOMENT.

**Puzzle 69**

SHUN IDLENESS. IT IS THE RUST THAT ATTACHES ITSELF TO THE MOST BRILLIANT METALS.

**Puzzle 70**

IF I TAKE CARE OF MY CHARACTER, MY REPUTATION WILL TAKE CARE OF ITSELF.

**Puzzle 71**

HE WHO ESTABLISHES HIS ARGUMENT BY NOISE AND COMMAND SHOWS THAT HIS REASON IS WEAK.

**Puzzle 72**

WHENEVER I FEEL LIKE EXERCISING, I LIE DOWN UNTIL THE FEELING PASSES.

**Puzzle 73**

TRUST YOUR OWN INSTINCT. YOUR MISTAKES MIGHT AS WELL BE YOUR OWN INSTEAD OF SOMEONE ELSE'S.

**Puzzle 74**

THE ONLY PEOPLE WHO LISTEN TO BOTH SIDES OF A FAMILY QUARREL ARE THE NEXT DOOR NEIGHBOURS.

**Puzzle 75**

ALL THE BEAUTIFUL SENTIMENTS IN THE WORLD WEIGH LESS THAN A SINGLE LOVELY ACTION.

**Puzzle 76**

THERE'S NOTHING IN THE MIDDLE OF THE ROAD BUT YELLOW STRIPES AND DEAD ARMADILLOS.

**Puzzle 77**

THE GEM CANNOT BE POLISHED WITHOUT FRICTION, NOR MAN PERFECTED WITHOUT TRIALS.

**Puzzle 78**

REMEMBER, WHEN THE PEACOCK STRUTS HIS STUFF HE SHOWS HIS BACKSIDE TO HALF THE WORLD.

**Puzzle 79**

LACK OF WILL POWER AND DRIVE CAUSE MORE FAILURES THAN LACK OF INTELLIGENCE AND ABILITY.

**Puzzle 80**

BELIEVE IT OR NOT, ONCE UPON A TIME, ALL MEMBERS OF THE FAMILY HAD BREAKFAST TOGETHER.

**Puzzle 81**

IF YOU WILL SPEND MORE TIME SHARPENING THE AXE, YOU'LL SPEND LESS TIME CHOPPING WOOD.

**Puzzle 82**

THE WORSHIP MOST ACCEPTABLE TO GOD COMES FROM A THANKFUL AND CHEERFUL HEART.

**Puzzle 83**

THE LAND OF MILK AND HONEY HAS ITS DRAWBACKS. YOU CAN GET KICKED BY A COW AND STUNG BY A BEE.

**Puzzle 84**

WHEN A MAN SEES THE HANDWRITING ON THE WALL, THERE IS PROBABLY A CHILD IN THE FAMILY.

**Puzzle 85**

PERSONALITY CAN OPEN DOORS BUT ONLY CHARACTER CAN KEEP THEM OPEN.

**Puzzle 86**

GOD'S TOMORROW WILL BE BETTER THAN ANY YESTERDAY YOU HAVE EVER KNOWN.

**Puzzle 87**

FOUR THINGS DO NOT COME BACK; THE SPOKEN WORD, THE SHOT ARROW, THE PAST LIFE AND THE NEGLECTED OPPORTUNITY.

**Puzzle 88**

I FINALLY KNOW WHAT DISTINGUISHES MAN FROM THE BEASTS: FINANCIAL WORRIES.

**Puzzle 89**

NO PASSION SO EFFECTUALLY ROBS THE MIND OF ALL ITS POWERS OF ACTING AND REASONING AS FEAR.

**Puzzle 90**

BRAVERY IS THE CAPACITY TO PERFORM PROPERLY EVEN WHEN SCARED HALF TO DEATH.

**Puzzle 91**

OPPORTUNITY IS MISSED BY MOST PEOPLE BECAUSE IT IS DRESSED IN OVERALLS AND LOOKS LIKE WORK.

# Index

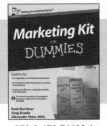
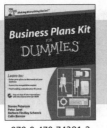
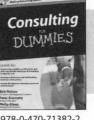
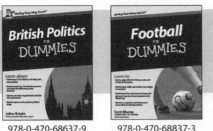
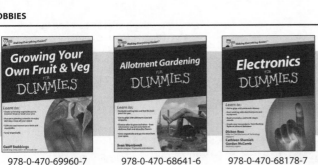

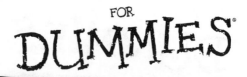

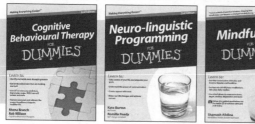
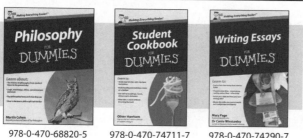
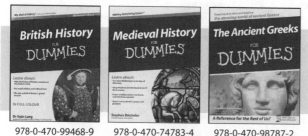

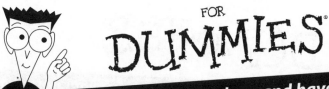

## FOR DUMMIES®

### The easy way to get more done and have more fun

---

## LANGUAGES

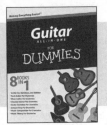

978-0-470-68815-1
UK Edition

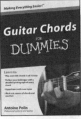

978-0-7645-5193-2

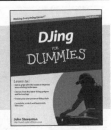

978-0-471-77270-5

Art For Dummies
978-0-7645-5104-8

Bass Guitar For Dummies, 2nd Edition
978-0-470-53961-3

Christianity For Dummies
978-0-7645-4482-8

Criminology For Dummies
978-0-470-39696-4

Forensics For Dummies
978-0-7645-5580-0

German For Dummies
978-0-7645-5195-6

Hobby Farming For Dummies
978-0-470-28172-7

Index Investing For Dummies
978-0-470-29406-2

Knitting For Dummies, 2nd Edition
978-0-470-28747-7

Music Theory For Dummies
978-0-7645-7838-0

Piano For Dummies, 2nd Edition
978-0-470-49644-2

Physics For Dummies
978-0-7645-5433-9

Schizophrenia For Dummies
978-0-470-25927-6

Sex For Dummies, 3rd Edition
978-0-470-04523-7

Sherlock Holmes For Dummies
978-0-470-48444-9

Solar Power Your Home
For Dummies, 2nd Edition
978-0-470-59678-4

The Koran For Dummies
978-0-7645-5581-7

Wine All-in-One For Dummies
978-0-470-47626-0

Yoga For Dummies, 2nd Edition
978-0-470-50202-0

## MUSIC

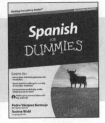

978-0-470-48133-2

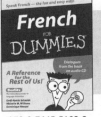

978-0-470-66603-6
Lay-flat, UK Edition

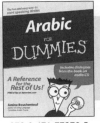

978-0-470-66372-1
UK Edition

## SCIENCE & MATHS

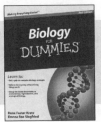

978-0-470-59875-7

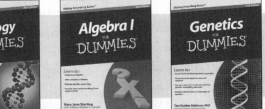

978-0-470-55964-2

978-0-470-55174-5

19546 (p3)

---

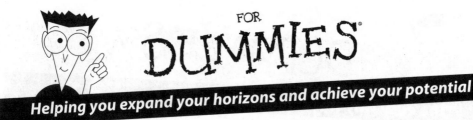
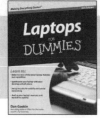
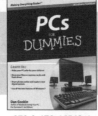
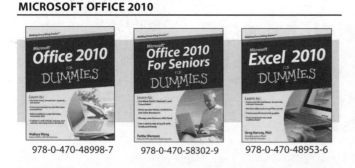